Solving
the
Health Care
Problem

Solving
the
Health Care
Problem

*How Other Nations Succeeded
and Why the United States Has Not*

PAMELA BEHAN

State University of New York Press

Published by
State University of New York Press, Albany

© 2006 State University of New York

For information, address State University of New York Press,
194 Washington Avenue, Suite 305, Albany, NY 12210-2384

Production by Judith Block
Marketing by Michael Campochiaro

Library of Congress Cataloging-in-Publication Data

Behan, Pamela.
  Solving the health care problem : how other nations succeeded and why
the United States has not / Pamela Behan.
    p. cm.
  Includes bibliographical references and index.
  ISBN 0-7914-6837-2 (hardcover : alk. paper)
  1. Medical policy—United States. 2. Right to health care—United States.
3. Medical care, Cost of—Government policy—United States. 4. Insurance,
Health—United States. I. Title.
  [DNLM: 1. Health Policy—United States. 2. Health Services Accessibility—
United States. 3. Health Care Costs—United States. 4. Insurance, Health—
United States.   WA 540 AA1 B39s 2006]
RA395.A3B44 2006
362.1—dc22

ISBN-13: 978-0-7914-6837-1 (hardcover : alk. paper)

10 9 8 7 6 5 4 3 2 1

Contents

TABLES   vii

INTRODUCTION   ix
    The Research Question   ix
    Explanations from the Literature   x
    The Research Method   xix
    The Book   xxx

CHAPTER 1. WHAT CAN THIS APPROACH TELL US?   1

CHAPTER 2. CANADA   5
    Historical Influences and Legacies   5
    Canadian Health Care Reform Initiatives   16
    Theoretical Explanations and Canadian Health Policy   30

CHAPTER 3. AUSTRALIA   33
    Historical Influences and Legacies   33
    Australian Health Care Reform Initiatives   38
    Theoretical Explanations and Australian Health Policy   53

CHAPTER 4. THE UNITED STATES   59
    Historical Influences and Legacies   60
    Division, Delay, and Private Entrenchment   67
    U.S. Health Care Reform Initiatives   72
    Theoretical Explanations and U.S. Health Policy   85

CHAPTER 5. A SECOND, SYSTEMATIC APPROACH 91
    The Theoretical Implications of the Three National Studies 91
    A Systematic Comparative Historical Method 97
    The Qualitative Comparative Analysis 99
    Results 107

CHAPTER 6. CONCLUSIONS 111
    Theoretical Conclusions from the Traditional Study 111
    What the Systematic Study Adds 115
    So What? 117
    Limitations to the Study 119
    Directions for Future Research 120

APPENDICES 123
    Appendix A. The Selection of Cases 123
    Appendix B. A Typology of Health Policy Outcomes 126
    Appendix C. The Choice of Causal Factors 132
    Appendix D. The Final Sixteen Factors and "Constants" 137
    Appendix E. A Short Introduction to Qualitative Comparative
        Analysis 138
    Appendix F. Tables used in the Qualitative Comparative
        Analysis 141

NOTES 145

BIBLIOGRAPHY 149

INDEX 163

Tables

1. Causation and Mills' Methods according to Ragin (1987)   xxi

2. Mills' and Ragin's Models of Causation Expanded   108

3. Case Typification by Outcome: Public (P), Decommodifying (D)   129

4. Case Outcome Types, Categorized by Citizens and Services
   Covered   130

5. Sixteen-Factor Summary Table   135

6. Summary Table of the Six Emergent Factors by Outcome Type   136

7. Representative Idealized Truth Table with Three Factors   139

8. Truth Table for the Six Emergent Factors (condensed)   141

9. Truth Table for the Two Sufficient Factors   142

10. Truth Table for the Four Necessary Conditions   142

11. Summary Table by Nation   143

Introduction

THE RESEARCH QUESTION

Of all the industrialized democracies, the United States is the only one that does not provide its citizens with either a national health care system or national health insurance (NHI) (Steinmo and Watts 1995: 330; Starr 1982: 288).[1] More specifically, the United States is the only such nation that allows its citizens to go entirely without care for lack of funds or to go bankrupt as a result of health problems (Navarro 1992: vii). This book presents the results of an investigation into this unique characteristic of U.S. national policy.

This introduction describes the theoretical and methodological approach of that study and is intended for readers interested in such particulars. Other readers may wish to begin with chapter 1, using the introduction only to answer specific questions about the study not addressed in the regular chapters.

The body of the introduction begins with a description of the main theories of cross-national difference in the welfare state literature. This is followed by an analysis of weaknesses in the literature that this study was designed to address. The theoretical approach of the study is then described, including the premises used by the author to guide both data gathering and the categorization of outcomes for analysis.

The second section of the introduction describes the method used to study the research question. It begins with an analysis of the research question, which is argued to be comparative, qualitative, and historical in nature, requiring a comparative historical methodological approach. Dilemmas presented by such methods and the major strategies available to address them are then cited and explained. The logic behind the choice of nations for comparison to the United States is described, followed by an account of the sources of data utilized. Finally, a short description of the rest of the book is provided.

EXPLANATIONS FROM THE LITERATURE

Since the 1950s, five central theoretical approaches have been used to account for national variance in social welfare policies such as health care. Three of these gained wide acceptance in spite of major limitations, most likely because they do not challenge the fairness of current arrangements. These theories are now recognized as relevant but limited in their usefulness on such questions.

Mainstream Approaches

Economic development has long been recognized as relevant to national welfare states. Until the early 1980s, convergence or logic-of-industrialization theory was the predominant explanation among social scientists for the emergence of national welfare state policies. This theory posits that all industrializing countries go through similar stages, which will eventually lead to convergence in national policies, including similar welfare state policies. However, convergence theory could never account satisfactorily for major policy differences among industrially advanced nations. In the early 1980s, studies increasingly challenged its predictions, focusing attention instead on the need for political and class variables (Quadagno 1987). Recently, globalization and welfare state retrenchment in a number of nations have revived interest in this theory, but available evidence still does not support its predictions (Olsen 2002; Banting 1997).

A second, widely recognized factor in welfare state determination has been national values or culture. The cultural theoretical approach regards policy differences among industrial nations as a matter of national political preferences, expressed through the democratic process (Fuchs 1986; Fein 1986; Ginzberg 1977; Lipset 1989). However, this theory could never explain the major discrepancies found between the policies preferred by the public and the policies actually adopted. Cultural theory came under challenge as studies increasingly emphasized the importance of conflicting values within national cultures, because it ignores the role of actors and power in asserting one version over another as a basis for policy (Blendon 1989; Olsen 2002; Navarro 1989; Parenti 1986; Stanfield 1979).

By the end of the 1980s, cross-national variance in welfare state policies was being explained in terms of three other theoretical traditions; one of these emphasizes interest-group competition, while the other two stress the organization of the central state and the strength of social democratic forces (Quadagno 1987). The first of these, pluralist or interest-group theory, is widely accepted within the United States but has proved to be of limited value on this question.

Pluralist theory notes that political actors in some nations, such as the United States, mobilize around specialized interests rather than along class lines (McConnell 1966; Polsby 1984; Dahl 1986:246). Pluralists then attribute the effectiveness of such organized groups in influencing legislation to cultural or strategic factors (Starr 1982; Marmor and Christianson 1982). However, this attribution rests on the presumption that all interest groups are relatively equal in power; as such, it cannot account for the enormous differences in their impact on legislation and policy. For instance, the coalition of organized physicians, businesses, and insurance companies regularly opposing national health insurance legislation has been extremely influential, but the advocates of such policy, in spite of broad public support, have not (Hirshfield 1970; Starr 1982; Blendon 1989). Explaining such differences in power is clearly central to answering our question, making pluralist theory, along with convergence and cultural theory, of limited usefulness here.

However, some quite useful information has been gained from comparative pluralist studies; it appears that pluralist political dynamics replace class-based dynamics only under particular national conditions. Countries that organize along interest-group lines have been noted to be those with weak or fragmented class organization, and political systems in which power is divided rather than centralized (Pampel 1994). For instance, if a nation's working class is divided, as it has been in the United States, its opponents are likely to pursue policies that exacerbate those divisions, and where the fragmentation of state power creates multiple points at which legislation may be blocked or altered, such policies are likely to be adopted as compromises. Over time, such policies would logically render politicians and bureaucrats less accountable to the shared interests of working-class citizens and more accountable to narrower interests. Political success would then become tied to the pursuit of narrow interests, creating a political system organized along interest-group lines.

The political and class conditions that result in such a system appear to be important variables to examine in accounting for U.S. policy exceptionalism. Fortunately, these factors are the same ones emphasized by the two remaining theoretical approaches.

Political Institutional Theories

Institutional theories stress the role of political and state institutions in determining and shaping welfare state policies. This is a multifaceted approach, which may emphasize the structure of state institutions, initiatives taken by autonomous officials, or the effects of policy legacies (Skocpol and Amenta 1986; Huber et al. 1993). It may focus on the activities of the state bureaucracy or the relative timing of institutional changes such as democratization or bureaucratization (Quadagno 1987). Its theorists may explore constitutionally mandated or evolved institutional processes and how they affect the strategic environment in which policy is decided (Huber et al. 1993; Immergut 1992b). Finally, they may seek to identify and compare the interactive effects of presidential/congressional and parliamentary systems, federal and unitary systems, bicameral and unicameral legislatures, and two-party and multiparty systems, along with those of electoral rules, the apportioning of representation, and regional and ideological coalitions (Olsen 2002:142–61; Banting 1997:281–84).

How would institutional theories explain U.S. exceptionalism? The United States differs significantly from other nations in its central state structures; specifically, its organization as a federation of states and the federal separation of powers are most often mentioned in this regard. These American constitutional structures are considered to be antagonistic to welfare state policies. The organization of the American national government as a federation of states has been theorized to slow the growth of its welfare state by weakening the power of the central government and its managers and by reducing support for welfare state policies at the national level (Gray 1991:7–11). Similarly, the constitutional division of the power to initiate and approve policy between the president and two branches of Congress, which may represent different parties or different ideological branches of one party, allows political minorities to veto welfare state legislation by providing multiple critical points where leverage can be applied and legislation stopped or altered (Steinmo and Watts 1995). The repeated failures of majority-supported legislation under this system then reduce majority solidarity by making the pursuit of narrower interests more strategic and winnable.

As would be expected with such a political legacy, the influence of private-sector interests on legislation and policy has been argued to be relatively greater in the United States than in other nations (Starr 1982; Starr and Immergut 1987:239; Laham 1993). The connection between this influence and institutional structure is described by Ellen Immergut's work, which describes how institutional procedures select the groups whose views will be represented and shape demands by structuring the strategic environment (1992b; see also Dahl 1956:137). U.S. national health policies are argued to have created both a new, bureaucratic health care model (Morone 1993) and a uniquely market-dominated policy legacy (Stone 1993).

Constitutionally mandated and evolved electoral processes in the United States are also relevant to political institutional accounts of U.S. exceptionalism. The winner-take-all system in the United States, for instance, is argued to have determined our two-party system, by preventing third parties from effectively influencing policy (Lipset 1967:335–38; Seligman 1987:95; Lipset 1989:201–05). The two-party system, combined with a lack of responsible party government, then led to the situation in which NHI's most powerful advocate, organized labor, was primarily affiliated for most of the last century with the same political party that represented the southern white elite. That elite has been shown to have used its position within the Democratic Party and the congressional seniority system to prevent the passage of universal national welfare state programs, which would have destabilized the racist southern labor system (Quadagno 1994).

Several studies have suggested bureaucratic-related barriers to NHI in the United States, including the early introduction of universal suffrage (Hanneman and Hollingsworth 1992), the resulting form, impact, and political party connections of bureaucracies (Weir and Skocpol 1983, 1986; Olsen 2002:158–59), and the electoral, congressional, and legislative response to the resulting patronage-oriented bureaucratic systems (Steinmo and Watts 1995). More recent studies have suggested other political institutional barriers, including the overrepresentation of rural America in the Senate, the coalition of U.S. racial and religious conservatives (Banting 1997:281–84), the impact of institutional processes and rules on U.S. political parties (Maioni 1998), the constraining effect on organized labor of the health insurance policy legacy it helped create (Gottschalk 2000), and the interaction between electoral politics and the congressional committee system (Olsen 2002:146).

Social Democratic / Power Resources Theory

Power resources theorists,[2] in contrast, approach their subject from a class perspective. These theorists accept Karl Marx's premise that the working class is a subordinated class in a capitalist society and that the state is generally dominated by the capitalist class. Unlike instrumental or structural Marxists, however, these theorists regard political control of the democratic state as a viable strategy for workers engaged in the democratic class strug-- gle, with the state as the site of struggle (Korpi 1983). Power resources theorists regard strong welfare state policies as victories won over capital by organized workers and specify democratic politics as the primary mechanism through which labor is able to force such reforms. They note that it is usually a socialist or working-class political party that demands the implementation of such policies and, when in power, introduces them into law (Esping-Andersen 1990; Navarro 1989; Korpi 1983).[3] In explaining national welfare state differences, power resources theorists specifically call attention to the balance of politically useful resources controlled by the capitalist and working classes in a given society (Korpi 1985).

A variation in the literature on this theme suggests that progressive policy has sometimes been implemented under conservative leadership to quiet working-class agitation and prevent the development of effective political opposition (Navarro 1989; Piven and Cloward 1971, 1977).[4] Since this strategy is useless once effective political opposition has been organized, this variation has usually been applied either to industrializing states or to industrialized states such as the United States where the working class is exceptionally weak. One implication of this idea is that, in nations where labor has not overcome racial, gender, blue collar/white collar, or other divisions, capitalist actors should be able to design policy to exploit those divisions and obscure shared working-class interests.

How would power resources theory address U.S. exceptionalism? The United States is unique among industrialized nations in both the weakness of its labor movement and the lack of an effective socialist or working-class party (Navarro 1989). The "failure of socialism" in the United States has been variously attributed to characteristics of the American socialist movement or its supporters, the lack of a feudal heritage, the presence of a frontier, mass immigration, exceptional social mobility, particular political structures, and a unique national system of beliefs and values (Seligman 1987: 91–105). Whatever the cause of this weakness, there is little disagreement that a stronger labor movement or a mainstream labor party would have considerable impact on U.S. health care policies. Power resources theory would also call attention to specific attributes of that movement or party, such as the qualities of its leadership and organization or alliances with other classes (Korpi 1985). U.S. exceptionalism in health care policy may reflect unique qualities of the health care domain, which make comprehensive reform especially difficult in the absence of strong working-class resources for building and exercising power.

However, U.S. welfare state policy in general has been noted to favor market-dominated, means-tested programs with modest benefits (Esping-Andersen 1990). The only partial exceptions to this characterization of U.S. welfare state policy are the Social Security and Medicare programs.

The Social Security program is a publicly run old age pension program that is employment-related but not means-tested; it offers very real protection for former workers in old age but also reinforces the inequality of the marketplace with market-based eligibility standards and unequal benefits. It is redistributive and public but does not reduce worker dependence on the market; furthermore, it primarily redistributes income between generations and genders, rather than between income strata. This popular, nearly universal program is noted to have become law under a Democratic administration during the Great Depression, when working-class mobilization and labor militancy were at their height in this country (Navarro 1989). During this period, several policies initially advocated by American socialists became popular and were passed into law as part of the New Deal.

Medicare, the health insurance program for retirees closely based on the Social Security program, became law during an unusual period of overwhelming Democratic Party legislative as well as executive dominance. It should also be noted that the late 1960s, like the Depression era, was a time of political mobilization and militancy, although organized more around opposition to racism and imperialism than around social class. Perhaps as a result, Medicare is less universal and less public than Social Security; that is, it addresses the health needs of only one category of citizens and relies on a voluntary private market component for their medical coverage. Only Medicare's hospital insurance component is truly public. Although somewhat more class redistributive than Social Security, Medicare's redistributive effects are also mainly generational and gendered; both its voluntary medical insurance component and the large proportion of health care costs it requires retirees to pay prevent Medicare from reducing worker dependence upon the market.

From a power resources point of view, then, neither Social Security nor Medicare represents the success of decommodifying or class redistributive welfare state policies in the United States; they represent exceptions only as public, nonmeans-tested social insurance programs. Class theorists would argue that democratic politics was the means of winning these public policy reforms during times of unusual militancy and mobilization, while the specific provisions of both programs reflect the overall weakness of the working class in the United States. As a policy that includes, at the least, an expansion of the public realm and of worker rights through that realm, NHI may be exceptional in the United States because of its relevance to the class struggle and not its unique domain.

Political institutional and power resources theory appear to be the critical theoretical approaches to include in a study of this question. Notably, these theories appear to be potentially complementary rather than necessarily contradictory. For instance, if political institutional arrangements determine the types of issues that can succeed legislatively, one side in the democratic class struggle may be systematically favored over the other by those institutions, giving it more influence in policy decisions. Alternatively, it is possible that the class struggle shapes political institutions so that over time, the power resources controlled by opposing social classes determine the processes that create or limit policies.

Weaknesses in the Literature

The literature exploring this research question shows several gaps, which this study was designed to address. First, formal studies in this literature have been dominated by single theory approaches, which are easier to test but tend to discount the shifting and multidimensional nature of national welfare state policy dynamics. However, there is no overwhelming reason to presume that the same dynamic is always the dominant one in different times and places and good reason to fear that such a presumption may lead to misleading results. The existence of patterns or configurations of welfare state outcomes argues instead for the cumulative effects of multiple interdependent causal factors, with nonlinear, sequential, or interactive effects (Pierson 2000:809).

Second, the literature exploring U.S. health policy primarily involves studies of dynamics within the United States, rather than systematic comparison with other nations. However, national exceptionalism can only be established, by definition, in comparison with other nations; how that difference came to be is therefore a question for comparison with other nations as well. Without explicit comparison, no perspective can be gained on the uniqueness of processes within a single nation or on the differential impact of common factors under different national conditions.

Third, the literature on health care policy has tended to treat it as a separate issue, too specialized to be considered on the same grounds as other welfare state issues (Wilensky et al., 1987). This is perhaps a carryover from the specialized nature of medicine and the claims of medical specialists to legitimately dominate matters of health care. However, national health care policy, however complex, involves the same issues of class redistribution, decommodification,[5] entitlement, universal versus targeted citizen benefits, state centralization and market stratification as pensions, unemployment insurance, family allowances, housing assistance, and other social policies. There is no logical reason to exclude it from similar analysis and every reason to expect such analysis to be useful (Moran 2000; Clarke and McEldowney 2000; Blake and Adolino 2001).

Fourth, cross-national comparative studies of national health care policy have rarely used outcome measures appropriate for addressing such qualitative welfare state issues as who benefits from specific national expenditures or how well citizens are protected by them. There is a good deal of work yet to be done, therefore, in sorting out health policy dynamics around redistribution, decommodification, social rights, and other qualitative questions.

Finally, political struggles that involve class interests are rarely explored as such in American analyses. Social class is frequently ignored altogether, or proxies such as race are employed to "stand in" for class dynamics. Both of these strategies hinder clarity on welfare state issues that, if only by their redistributive properties, logically involve issues of class interest and competition. The assumption appears to be that, because politics are organized pluralistically in the United States, class dynamics are altogether absent here. However, that assumption should be logically treated as an empirical question, not a fact.

This study addresses these weaknesses by addressing U.S. health care policy as a qualitative, comparative welfare state issue and by explicitly considering multicausal or conjunctural causal dynamics, including those of social class.

Two Theoretical Premises

Any systematic study of this research question must take all of these theories into consideration. This study utilizes political institutional and class power factors as its main causal or explanatory variables, includes interest-group variables to test their relevance, and takes convergence and cultural theory into consideration in its choice of nations for comparison.

Two theoretical premises were formed early in this research and used to inform the data-gathering process. The first was that class power factors were necessary, but probably not sufficient, to answer this research question. This followed from the redistributive nature of the policy issue and the observation that, while working-class organization had started earlier and been at least as strong in the United States as in Canada or Australia, both the successes and the strength of the U.S. labor movement fell behind those of the other two nations over time. This suggested that some third factor or factors affected social democratic dynamics in the United States differently than in Canada or Australia.

The second theoretical premise was that political institutions might be the third factor that differentially affected class power dynamics in these nations. This followed from two empirical observations. One was that the battle for the right to collective bargaining took far longer in the United States than in Australia or Canada; the other was that U.S. labor found it necessary to abandon political tactics that were successful in both Australia and Canada. Logically, if unusually hostile political institutions in the United States had the power to counteract direct labor tactics and render most union strategies ineffective, U.S. social democratic dynamics would necessarily assume a different form than in nations where those tactics and strategies met with success. A relative lack of success could also prompt discouragement with working-class organization, explaining the loss of U.S. union strength over time.

The role of interest-group dynamics was then tentatively conceptualized as residual in relation to class issues; that is, where working-class political organizations are repeatedly blocked from achieving their goals, narrower forms of political organization might come to dominate welfare state issues. This would not necessarily mean that interest-group dynamics assume no importance at all for such issues in nations where working-class organization has been successful; it implies only that they would dominate outcomes less than where working-class organization was less successful. Empirically, interest-group activity may be capable of accommodating itself to a wide variety of class power arrangements.

Theoretically, then, this author approached her subject with the expectation that both political institutional theory and power resource theory might be relevant to the research question. Whether one might turn out to be determinant of the other, or the exact nature of the relations between theoretically relevant factors, was not presupposed.

THE RESEARCH METHOD

The Nature of the Research Question

The research question addressed in this study is comparative, qualitative, and historical in nature. As argued earlier, policy exceptionalism is by definition a comparative issue. The uniqueness of dynamics that result in unique national policy outcomes can only be understood with reference to the dynamics and outcomes of other nations.

It is also a qualitative question. Both quantitative and qualitative methods have been used to compare and explain national policy differences. However, since our query seeks to unravel the complex political and institutional dynamics around a specifiable national policy outcome, it requires close attention to the dynamics of numerous policy events, a qualitative process. Neither complex, interactive causal factors, nor the complex variable qualities of policy outcomes in different nations can be adequately measured and compared through quantitative measures (Ragin 1987; Orloff 1993).

A number of comparative qualitative approaches could be envisioned. However, national policy exceptionalism is also a historical issue. That is, the U.S. lack of national health insurance is exceptional because, over time, all other industrialized nations have adopted such protections, while the United States has not. The question of how other nations have managed to pass such legislation into law, and how it has been blocked in this country, must be answered with reference to the past. Furthermore, contemporary efforts can only be understood with reference to a nation's historical legacy; the costs "of adopting previously available alternatives" are drastically increased by social adaptation to existing policies and procedures (Pierson 2000:811). A historical comparative approach, therefore, was adopted.

Comparative Historical Dilemmas and Solutions

Comparative historical methods are as old and venerable as the social sciences themselves. Traditionally, such methods rely on historical accounts for their research material and on analytic logic for their results. Recently, several social scientists have clarified that logic, explored several potential weaknesses, and identified some ways of addressing these weaknesses (Tilly 1984; Skocpol 1984; Ragin 1987).

The first such weakness involves a failure to look beyond the possibility of a single, main cause for complex historical phenomena. According to Charles Ragin, this has followed from excessive reliance on John Stuart Mills' delineation of research strategies for generalizing from empirical observations when the experimental manipulation of variables is not feasible. Specifically, comparative historical studies have built on Mills' method of agreement and indirect method of difference ([1843] 1967).

The method of agreement argues that "if two or more instances of a phenomenon under investigation have only one of several possible causal circumstances in common, then the circumstance in which all the instances agree is the cause of the phenomenon of interest" (Ragin 1987:36). The investigator applies this method by identifying instances of an outcome (positive cases), then determining what factor invariably precedes this outcome; this factor is then identified as causal. The method of agreement is not a statistical technique; the factor must always precede the outcome of interest, or it is disqualified as the cause (Mills [1843] 1967; Ragin 1987).

However, this method only establishes correlation and may therefore lead to false or spurious conclusions. That is, a factor may be present in every positive case without being responsible for its outcome. Furthermore, as Ragin shows, this method logically leads to the rejection of true causal factors when any of several causal conditions may independently produce the outcome of interest. Under this pattern, called "multiple independent causation," each independent cause may be absent from some positive cases, and is thereby falsely rejected (1987).

Mills developed the indirect method of difference to check the results of the method of agreement. The investigator applies this method

TABLE 1.
CAUSATION AND MILLS' METHODS ACCORDING TO RAGIN (1987)

Patterns of Causation	Method of Agreement: Is the causal factor present in all positive cases?	Indirect Method of Difference: Is the causal factor absent from all negative cases?
Single Causation: (one necessary and sufficient factor)	yes	yes
Multiple Independent Causation: (multiple sufficient but not necessary factors, interchangeable in their effect)	no (a potential source of error)	yes
Conjunctural Causation: (multiple necessary but not sufficient factors, causal in combination)	yes	no (a potential source of error)

by identifying instances of the absence of the outcome of interest (nega-tive cases), then determining the presence or absence of the purported causal factor for each such case. The factor must be absent from all nega-tive cases to be supported as the cause of the phenomenon of interest. Again, the indirect method of difference is not a statistical technique; it requires perfect correlation to support a hypothesis (Mills [1843] 1967; Ragin 1987).

Unfortunately, this technique can also lead to false results. Specifi-cally, in the case of an outcome that actually results from the simultane-ous presence of two or more factors ("conjunctural causation"), the isolated presence of any of those factors in a negative case will cause the investigator to falsely reject them (Ragin 1987). Table 1 summarizes Ragin's arguments.

According to Ragin, then, the formal application of Mills' methods in comparative historical research will identify only single causes of out-comes; the researcher must be aware of the potential for multiple inde-pendent or conjunctural causation to avoid misleading results. Fourth and fifth steps, specifically testing for multiple independent and conjunctural causation, are logically indicated. Ragin (1987) has created a method for systematically carrying out these additional steps, beginning with the reduction of pertinent information to tables that list the causal factors and outcomes of interest as either present (1) or absent (0). Boolean algebra can then be used to check for multiple independent and conjunctural causation (Ragin 1987). This approach is called Qualitative Comparative Analysis (QCA) and is used in this study to supplement and systematically check the results of the traditional comparative historical analyses (Hicks 1994; Ragin 1987).

A second methodological weakness concerns a lack of agreement on identifying outcomes of interest. For instance, NHI programs have been implemented in different nations in multiple forms, and there is little agreement on what constitutes its essential elements. Some forms include all citizens, others include all resident citizens and noncitizens, and still others include only those resident citizens qualified by some criteria. So even if all social scientists were to agree that NHI is defined by the quality of universality, no agreement exists at present as to what constitutes universality. Similarly, even if we agree that NHI must, at a minimum, guarantee all citizens access to health care and protection from health care costs, there is no agreement as to what constitutes reasonable access or financial protection. Therefore, our outcome of interest, NHI, is a disputed rather than an easily identified and agreed upon phenomenon, and the designation of positive and negative cases can be expected to be controversial.

One solution to this dilemma is to use Tilly's distinction of different types as providing negative cases for each other (1984). That is, the qualities of interest in NHI programs can be delineated and used to distinguish different types of national health policy from among a range of nations, including the United States; cases with different types of outcomes can then be used as negative cases for one another. For example, instances of political initiatives resulting in national health policy addressing basic care for citizens poor enough to pass a means test ("residual" type outcomes) could be used as negative cases for those instances resulting in comprehensive public insurance for all citizens ("decommodifying" type outcomes), and vice versa. The causal factors correlated with each type of case can then be compared with one another.

This solution offers the advantage of allowing the researcher to specify what is found and then suggest and defend logical typifications of those findings, rather than to use and assert agreement on larger nominal categorizations, such as NHI, that are in dispute. This offers, in effect, a middle-range methodology for building middle-range theory.

The application of this method to a study investigating a single negative case, however, highlights a third weakness of comparative historical methods. Many possible causal factors are likely to be identified through the method of agreement, but too few negative cases may make it impossible to distinguish the causal from the spurious factors. This is notably the case with U.S. exceptionalism, where several of the factors that have been identified as important to the passage of NHI in other countries—types of state institutions, types of political parties, labor movements, national cultures, and so on—are either absent, considerably weaker, or appear qualitatively different in the United States (Steinmo and Watts 1995; Navarro 1989; Lipset 1989).

One solution is to expand our definition of cases to include time periods as well as countries, creating negative and positive cases within a single country at different times, as well as negative and positive cases within different countries at similar times (Orloff 1993; Skocpol 1984). This is probably the best single solution if our outcome of interest is a single phenomenon, easily identified and agreed upon as present or absent in a particular time and place.

When it is not, however, the solution to the second dilemma can be used in combination with this one. That is, qualitatively different types of programs passed at different times within the same country can be used as negative cases for one another, as well as for different types of programs passed in other nations (see Orloff 1993). This is the strategy used in this book.

The Choice of Nations

The choice of nations to be compared is another important decision in comparative historical research. The "most similar nations" strategy is recommended as providing controls on possible causal factors not targeted in a specific study (Ragin 1987: 47–48), especially if the nations are chosen to vary primarily on the targeted causal factors (Orloff 1993). That is, nations for comparison are chosen to provide: (1) a mixed group of positive and negative cases on the outcome of interest; (2) minimum variation on nontargeted potential causal factors; and (3) maximum variation on targeted potential causal factors. This logically limits the number of causal factors, identified through the method of agreement, that must be sorted out in a study through the use of negative cases and the indirect method of difference. Recent studies utilizing the "most similar" strategy include Blankenau (2001), O'Connor, Orloff, and Shaver (1999), Maioni (1998), Banting (1997), Boase (1996), and Ruggie (1996).

This selection strategy acknowledges and is motivated by the fact that, since the actual number of nations is limited, the ideal combination of national variations for definitive testing of all possible causal factors is generally not attainable (Ragin 1987). Specifically, the number of possible causes of a phenomenon found in most groups of nations is going to be greater than the opportunities provided by negative cases to eliminate spurious factors from consideration. Multiple independent or conjunctural causation, in particular, can only be ruled out through the presence of negative cases providing the maximum possible variety of combinations of targeted, but spurious, causal factors. Such variety is therefore essential but unlikely to occur without a careful selection of nations and targeted factors. The result of ignoring this fact is a literature replete with nondefinitive studies, which contribute to our understanding of dynamics but do not allow us to state categorically what is causal and what is not.

The question then becomes how to choose nations and design studies to (1) examine a limited number of causal factors; (2) allow a definitive testing of those causal factors targeted; and (3) contribute to the eventual, systematic testing of all possible causal factors, in order to collectively reach definitive theoretical conclusions. While many researchers appear to implicitly accept and use these criteria in selecting nations and designing their studies, the collective strategy requires more systematic specification and application. In her 1993 book, for instance, Orloff describes her study design quite carefully but addresses her choice of Britain and Canada for comparison with the United States quite briefly and in very general terms. She provides neither a systematic defense of the centrality of her grounds nor a systematic discussion of possible choices of nations by possible causal factors, leaving her readers with little sense of the specific logic or appropriateness of her choices. Just as comparative research strategies have been clarified recently, case selection strategies require clarification as well.

The choice of nations for comparison in this study is based on (1) the nature of the research question, (2) systematic consideration of all the possible causal factors identified in the literature, and (3) the theoretical approach proposed for this study. The nature of the research question, the explanation of a paradox (Ragin 1987:47), creates a special need to restrict the choice of nations to those that are similar to the United States in as many theoretically relevant ways as possible so that we may concentrate on the relevant dissimilarities. That is, addressing the exceptionality of a single nation puts particular constraints on the researcher to control as many potential causal factors as possible in their choice of other nations for comparison. Systematic consideration of all the possible causal factors identified in the literature allows us to emphasize nontargeted suggested causal factors in choosing "most similar" nations, in order to avoid skewing the choice of nations to influence our results. Finally, the chosen nations must be shown to be appropriate for a particular study. For instance, the nations chosen for this study through the previous step must vary sufficiently from the United States and from one another, in both the targeted causal factors and policy outcomes, to offer real potential for explaining health policy variability in general and U.S. exceptionality in particular.

The welfare state and U.S. health policy literatures were examined for possible causal factors for this study. The welfare state literature explores differences in national policies relevant to citizens' welfare, including pensions, unemployment and disability income, and health care insurance or provision. Comparative welfare state studies have identified a range of social, political, and economic factors as potentially causal, including industrialization, national affluence (per capita GDP), democratic political processes, social democratic party rule, trade union strength, the requirements of advanced capitalism, state institutions and elites, policy legacies, divisions in the economy and working class, Catholicism or Christian democratic rule, mass political protest, interest-group activity, micro and macro-economic context, and population aging (Skocpol and Amenta 1986; Quadagno 1987; Esping-Andersen and van Kersbergen 1992; Hicks and Misra 1993; Huber et al. 1993; Pampel 1994).

Studies specifically on health care policy in the United States have suggested the relevance of some factors in addition to those identified above. U.S. economists and sociologists of culture favor a national values explanation of health care policy variance among industrialized nations, expressed as political preferences through the electoral process (Fuchs 1986; Fein 1986; Ginzberg 1977; Lipset 1989). The sheer size of the U.S. population and landmass has been suggested as a barrier to reform, in that it tends to increase the interested actors in any complex reform and to inhibit the development of the solidarity necessary for redistributive policy reform (White 1995: 376). Finally, policy analyst Deborah Stone suggests that market legacies are critical to explaining U.S. health care policies (1993).

Utilizing the theoretical considerations first that we will not target in this study, we confine our search to nations that, like the United States, are urbanized, industrialized, and capitalist democracies. To control as much as possible for cultural values, we further confine our search to other English-founded nations, where a common English heritage can be expected to include a legal foundation in English common law (i.e., Durkheim's precontractual), as well as a shared conceptual framework in the English language. For the most part, customs, social arrangements, and cultural understandings relevant either to the political process or to the provision of medical care can be expected to be similar to those of the United States in another nation with a shared English heritage.

Some of the nontargeted factors do not help us distinguish between the English-speaking nations. For instance, neither the United Kingdom, the United States, Canada, Australia, nor New Zealand is predominantly Catholic, and none have strong Christian democratic parties.

Then, on one nontargeted and several targeted factors, the United States is the exception. Canada and Australia approximate the size of the landmass of the United States, but none of the other four nations contains more than one-fifth the U.S. population (Population Reference Bureau, 1995). Trade unions are considerably stronger in Australia, Canada, New Zealand, and the United Kingdom than in the United States (Navarro 1989). None of these nations shares the unique constitutional institutions of the United States; each uses a variation of the British parliamentary system known as responsible party, cabinet, or Westminster system of government. Possibly for that reason, none of the other nations exhibits the level of interest-group influence seen in the United States (Mulgan 1994:194). On these important population, class, institutional, and pluralistic factors, there is considerable variation between all the other English-founded nations and the United States.

The other suggested causal factors, both targeted and nontargeted, are more helpful in making our choices. Four of these nations share similar demographics, with 12 to 13 percent of the population over 65 years of age, and 21 to 23 percent under 15; the single exception is the United Kingdom, with 16 percent and 19 percent, respectively—a pattern common in Northern and Western Europe (Population Reference

Bureau, 1995). By Esping-Andersen's criteria, the United States, Australia, and Canada share dualistic economies, with a resulting division in the working class; Britain and New Zealand are less clear in this regard (1990). Canada and Australia, like the United States, are federations, but Britain and New Zealand are not. Furthermore, Canadian federalism creates a provincial-federal division of powers similar in some of its effects to the U.S. executive-legislative division of powers (Thorburn 1985). Australia, New Zealand, and the United Kingdom have strong national labor parties; the United States has no such party, while the New Democratic Party in Canada is relatively weak nationally and has only become of national significance in the past few decades (Christian and Campbell 1983). Finally, none of the other Anglo-Saxon nations matches the affluence of the United States, although Canada is close, followed by Australia, the United Kingdom, and New Zealand, in that order (Population Reference Bureau, 1995). By these demographic, economic, constitutional, and political criteria, Canada shares the most relevant characteristics with the United States, with Australia the next "most similar" nation.

Even the casual observer cannot help but note the similarities in the historical and cultural heritages of these three nations. All were primarily founded, settled, and dominated by England in their formative periods; all began as separate colonies in newly discovered continents, pioneered on the lands of native peoples who were permanently displaced; all remain primarily English speaking; and all are federal in form. The possibility that policy dynamics are also similar is supported by qualitative studies that have found strong parallels between the politics of the five "Anglo-Saxon" nations (Alford 1973; Mulgan 1994:30; Marsh 1995:9, 12, 54).

Recent studies assist us in checking the appropriateness of these choices with reference to policy outcomes. We would expect truly similar nations to exhibit many policy similarities, and recent research has indeed identified distinct policy patterns among nations' welfare state policies that support this choice of nations.

Esping-Andersen's *Three Worlds of Welfare Capitalism* (1990) identifies three types of welfare states from data on 18 affluent industrialized nations, using measures of three variable characteristics of welfare states; these qualities are decommodification, stratification, and the public-private mix.[6] The first measures policies' effects upon the ability of citizens to live independently of the market, the second measures policies' effects upon status or class stratification, and the third captures the role of the market in a nation's welfare state. Based on measures of these three characteristics, Esping-Andersen finds three types of welfare states. Conservative welfare states, exemplified by Austria, France, Germany and Italy, grew within strong, authoritarian state regimes that adopted corporatist mechanisms. These states have preserved status differentials by attaching social rights and benefit levels to class and status (1990: 27). Social democratic regimes, exemplified by Norway, Sweden, and Denmark, began as liberal regimes but were altered through political struggle over control of the democratic state. These states have partially decommodified their citizens' labor through universal public programs, with services and benefits for all at middle-class levels (1990: 27–28). It is Esping-Andersen's third type, liberal welfare states, that concerns us here.

Liberal welfare states, exemplified by Australia, Canada, and the United States, are distinguished by minimal decommodification, dualistic programs, and market domination of the public-private mix (Esping-Andersen 1990: 26–27). This group offers only modest social insurance or universal programs, with state programs designed to encourage the private market, and only stigmatized, means-tested public assistance programs provided for those unable to compete successfully in the labor market. The consequence is a division, or "class-political dualism," between the majority of citizens and state-welfare recipients (1990:26–27). Esping-Andersen's findings suggest both a reference group and an analytic framework for the consideration of U.S. health care policy. They also support the choice of Australia and Canada as the nations most similar to the United States. In particular, the effect of policy feedbacks or legacies (Heclo 1974) increases the probability that nations with similar, well-established welfare state policies will develop similar political and bureaucratic institutions, issues, and interested parties, relative to those of other nations.

Sufficient variability in our theoretical factors of interest and health policy outcomes among the United States, Canada, and Australia also can be readily established. As mentioned above, Canada and Australia share the characteristics of stronger trade unions, parliamentary or responsible party government, and weaker interest-group activity than the United States. In contrast to Australia, however, Canada exhibits a more effective federal division of state power, a much weaker labor party, and more economic affluence. On all these possible causal factors, Canada falls between Australia and the United States.

However, Australia's NHI policy is considerably less comprehensive, generous, and universal than Canada's, making it more like the United

States on health policy outcome. The public/private mix in the Australian NHI program is also more like that of the United States than Canada's, where no role for commercial insurance interests was preserved (Gray 1991). Finally, Australia dismantled NHI after its initial passage and implementation, then reinstated it; this political ambivalence appears closer to the U.S. failure to pass NHI at all than Canada's unanimous passage and subsequent widespread support of NHI (Gray 1984, 1987). On health policy outcomes, then, Australia appears to fall between Canada and the United States.

On both the targeted causal factors and health policy outcomes, then, these three nations offer considerable variation. In addition, the direction of the most notable national differences in causal factors and outcomes appears contrary to theory and is therefore unlikely to reveal a simple linear relation. Instead, these findings suggest either the independent importance of more than one causal factor (multiple independent causation) or multiple interactive causal factors (conjunctural causation). This choice of nations appears appropriate for clarifying the dynamics of national health policy determination in the United States.

Sources of Data

Most of the facts in this book are taken from secondary sources. Where readily available, primary materials have been used to supplement this secondary material. While many other primary sources are undoubtedly available, most would have required a great deal of time and expense to utilize. Secondary sources are a reliable type of research data, however, as long as the researcher remains aware of their limitations and takes a few precautions.

One limitation of secondary sources is their tendency to select the material included on the basis of the theory being explored or the story being told. For instance, a study exploring the effects of federalism on health care policy could not be expected to include the relevant material on class politics or legislative dynamics needed for this study. For that reason, secondary sources were sought out that explained health policy from as many theoretical viewpoints as possible for each of the three countries.

A second problem with secondary sources is that they often rely on other secondary sources for information; in this process, interpretations may become indistinguishable from facts to the reader. For that reason, secondary sources based on predominantly primary source material were sought out and used as much as possible. In addition, critical facts obtained from secondary sources were double-checked whenever possible, using primary material when available.

Initially targeted political institutional factors included federal or subfederal responsibility for health care, federal/subfederal division of powers, responsible party government or separation of powers at the federal level, proportional representation or winner-take-all elections, multiparty or two-party political systems, and policy legacies. Initially targeted power resources factors included market legacies, politically unified or divided business interests, politically organized business groups, labor party strength and unity, and trade union strength, unity, and political activity. Initially targeted interest-group factors included politically unified or divided physicians, politically active physicians, unified or divided health care consumers, and politically organized consumers.

The qualities of interest used to typify policy outcomes initially included amounts and types of state involvement, inclusion or exclusion of private insurance companies, the percent of citizens covered, labor market-related qualifications for citizen inclusion, comprehensiveness of health care coverage, separate health care arrangements for those relying on state insurance and those paying extra, required patient copayments, the allowance of "extra billing" (billing of patients for amounts beyond those paid for by the insurance system), and contributory or tax-based financing. For both causal factors and outcomes, alteration of these initial categories proved necessary in order to fully capture all potentially significant variations in the data.

THE BOOK

Because it addresses a topic of considerable public interest, this book has been designed to be useable by nonspecialist readers. To that end, specialized theoretical and methodological discussions have been limited for the most part to the introduction and chapter 5; chapter 1 is provided as an alternative introduction to the topic and study.

Chapters 2, 3, and 4 focus on the individual nations of the study, combining descriptions of their relevant histories with traditional historical analyses of their paths to NHI success or failure. Chapter 5 then draws the relevant theoretical strands together in a more elaborated form and presents the Qualitative Comparative Analysis (QCA) with its results.

Finally, chapter 6 describes the study's overall conclusions in layman's terms.

More specific information on QCA and the analysis, which may interest more specialized readers, may be found in the appendices. Scholars interested in the original data base assembled by the author for the QCA will find it in the author's dissertation (Behan 2000).

CHAPTER 1

What Can This Approach Tell Us?

The purpose of this book is to help answer the question of why the United States does not guarantee its citizens access to health care or protect them from its costs. There are lots of reasonable-sounding answers to that question, but since many of them contradict one another, they cannot all be correct. This book takes the approach that we can get not only a correct answer but also the most useful answer to this question by centering our attention on the fact that all other industrialized democracies protect their citizens in this way. That is, the United States is the only democratic nation wealthy enough to afford universal health insurance that has not created such a program. In this area of "health security," the United States is the exception—the international standout—and the question this book addresses is, "Why?"

What would be a useful answer to this question, and how should we go about finding one? A useful answer, it seems to me, would be one that helps us solve the very real human problems associated with the question. In this case, that includes the shortened length and quality of life experienced by Americans who have health problems and no health insurance, who stay in jobs they hate because they cannot afford to lose their health benefits or who lose everything they have worked for to an expensive illness or accident. It includes the despair experienced by adults who cannot secure needed care for a beloved child, spouse, or parent and the poverty borne by those who use up every asset they have trying to help a loved one. It includes the helplessness felt by dedicated health professionals who struggle to get their patients the care they need yet regularly find themselves treating the chronic or terminal results of health care neglect. Finally, it includes the frustration experienced by those politicians, civil

1

servants, and citizen activists who have struggled in vain for decades to negotiate and pass legislative solutions to these problems.

What kind of answer is likely to help us solve such problems? It seems to me that we cannot find such an answer by looking only within the United States. Certainly we can learn much in that way about how solutions have been blocked in this country, about which groups and types of individuals have fought the creation of solutions, and about who makes profits or gains power from keeping things as they are. But none of that information really tells us how to deal with these obstacles. In contrast, we might learn much by looking at how other nations have managed to create solutions, what obstacles they faced in doing so, how they handled those obstacles, and how well their solutions worked. In other words, our difficulties may not be as unique as we think, but we cannot know without learning about other nations' experiences.

This book therefore takes a comparative and historical approach to its question. The comparative is to help us put the obstacles to health security in the United States in perspective, and to give us some idea of what we might have to do differently to solve these problems as other nations have. The historical approach is necessary because all the nations that have solved these problems acted to solve them at some point in the past, and knowledge of the conditions under which they were able to do so may be essential to similar successes in the United States.

What factors must such an approach include? First of all, it will require us to pay attention to any factors that may have shaped the problem differently in the United States than in other nations. This step may be simplified somewhat by choosing nations for comparison that resemble the United States in as many relevant ways as possible. For instance, Canada and Australia are the nations that most closely resemble the United States historically, culturally, politically, economically, and demographically. (For details, see "The Choice of Nations" in the introduction.) We can then concentrate on the factors that represent national differences to explain health policy differences among those nations.

Second, such an approach will require us to consider the class forces and interest groups that work for and against such public solutions, comparing their relative activity in other nations to our own. Class-based explanations regard protective legislation as victories for working-class citizens, which may be won in two ways. One is when workers organize powerfully enough to win control of government and pass such legislation themselves; the other is when a conservative government, threatened by such organization, passes such legislation to quiet worker agitation and prevent a loss of political control. Class theorists would therefore tend to explain the lack of U.S. health care protection by the relative weakness of the organized working class in the United States.

In contrast, pluralist or interest-group theorists focus on the power of groups organized around numerous specialized interests. They would tend to explain American exceptionalism by the relative strength of the highly visible coalition of interest groups that regularly oppose U.S. public health insurance. This point of view is supported by the tendency in the United States to think that the visibility of interest-group activities means that class, or social democratic, activities are irrelevant to our politics and policies. However, such factors have turned out to be quite important in explaining other welfare state policy differences across groups of nations including the United States, so we cannot safely assume that class factors do not matter here; they may simply be less visible or take a different form.

Third, such an approach will require us to gather information on the factors that may affect a democracy's responsiveness to class and interest-group activities, including its ability to agree and act upon specific political solutions to problems. There are many features of American government that may be important here. For instance, we are a federation of states, our Constitution deliberately divides power among executive, legislative, and judicial branches of government, and our election rules award everything to the winners, rather than proportioning representation by relative support. In addition, traditions within the House and Senate have divided the power to legislate between numerous powerful committees and individuals. A number of studies have suggested ways in which these arrangements may affect specific types of legislation, for instance, by allowing organized minorities to repeatedly block broadly based programs.

This study therefore begins with histories of the three nations, describing their political, class, medical, and health policy development, and the activities of political parties and organized groups pertaining to health policy. Each of these three chapters concludes with an analysis of the factors that appear to have been most relevant to that nation's health policy development. Chapter 5 pulls those explanatory strands together in a more comparative form, then checks the results by using even more detailed information in a systematic analysis, designed to avoid investigator bias. The results suggest that four specific conditions are necessary in these nations for progress to be made towards national health insurance; one of these has never been met by the United States. In addition, they suggest that either of two other conditions would be sufficient for such progress; neither of these has occurred in the United States. The final chapter then describes the study's conclusions in layman's terms, including the changes that may be needed to solve the problems of health care access and protection from its costs in the United States.

CHAPTER 2

Canada

Canada's national health insurance is characterized by its federal form, popularity, stability, and bipartisan support. Each province runs its own program, which must adhere to five coordinating principles to qualify for partial commonwealth funding. Canadian Medicare has enjoyed great stability due to its high level of public support and the consequent backing of all major political parties.

Canadian NHI has had a relatively smooth political history, although it was instituted quite late by international standards. Early Canadian health care policy was characterized by widely varying provincial policy experiments, which precipitated incremental changes toward a coordinated program at the commonwealth level. Canadian governments successfully weathered organized medicine's resistance to NHI in several provinces, insisting on a public right to limit professional prerogatives and profits.

HISTORICAL INFLUENCES AND LEGACIES

The first colonies in what is now Canada were not English at all, but French. The French Canadian legacy differentiates Canada from Australia and the United States in some ways potentially important to this work, and therefore will be explored in some depth.

The lands that became Arcadia (Nova Scotia) and New France (Quebec) were first claimed by France in 1534, with the first successful settlements begun at Port Royal in 1605, the city of Quebec in 1608, and Montreal in 1642; however, these colonies were then largely neglected. New France suffered a lack of steady support from either French merchants or the French court and was further plagued by competition from

5

English fur traders and involvement in the losing war of the Huron and Algonquin tribes against the Iroquois, allies of the Dutch in New York. The colony's fur trade was effectively disrupted, expansion prevented, and the settlements nearly lost by 1661, when France finally regained a strong position in Europe and an interest in expansion abroad. Even then, Arcadia had no immediate commercial prospects and received assistance from France only when its strategic position on the coast became important for the struggle with England over dominance of the New World. Nevertheless, both Arcadia and New France grew and prospered, along with a feudal agricultural system and the influence of the Catholic Church in the area (McInnis 1959:1–97).

However, the English colonies to the south also grew, and competition between English settlers and French fur traders for domination of the interior of the continent eventually resulted in war. Arcadia was lost to the English in 1713, but France fortified Louisburg, on Cape Breton Island, and continued hostilities over control of the area until 1755. In the end, the French Arcadian community was ordered to take an oath of allegiance to England, and upon its refusal, was rounded up and forcibly deported. Delays and shipwrecks resulted in families being broken up and the Arcadians widely scattered; as a result, Nova Scotia effectively lost its French community and character (McInnis 1959:98–114).

New France was lost to the English at the battle of the Plains of Abraham, ratified by the Treaty of Paris in 1763. With no other French strongholds in the area, the English were more generous in their occupation of New France than they had been in Arcadia. Local laws and taxes were allowed to continue unchanged, and the free exercise of the Catholic religion and security of property were promised to the inhabitants. Although changes in the laws were later made, including the exclusion of Catholics from public office, the French community in Quebec was allowed to maintain its language and customs, prospered, and with its high birth rate, continued to grow under English governance (McInnis 1959:115–39). This history of settlement and conquest is responsible for the dual cultural legacy of Canada and for the dynamic of French Canadian resistance to English Canadian dominance and control, including Quebec's leadership of provincial resistance to commonwealth domination.

The first health care institutions in Canada were therefore organized by French Catholic religious orders in New France, which imported the institutions of seventeenth-century France for the charitable care of the sick poor. Their patients included large numbers of Native Americans and new immigrants, who suffered particularly from periodic epidemics of smallpox, typhus, yellow fever, cholera, and influenza (Abbott 1931). A nun in Quebec recorded the effects of a 1650 smallpox epidemic in which the hospital's wards could not contain all the cases, so many sick Native Americans had to be housed in bark huts on an adjoining piece of land (Gibb 1855). Later epidemics were more likely to include large numbers of Irish immigrants, who often arrived on ships already plagued by disease. Many nuns and physicians died in these epidemics, which gradually abated over time as a result of sanitation efforts and vaccinations (Abbott 1931).

Most medical care in New France was, however, given by private or salaried practitioners in their patients' homes. Military or commercially sponsored immigrant groups invariably included a company surgeon; as a royal colony in the 1660s, New France was provided with salaried midwives and physicians to provide care to the colonists. Physicians in charge of the hospitals were apparently chosen by the nuns, but salaried by France. Other physicians, apothecaries, midwives, and barber-surgeons immigrated and made their own arrangements; at least one physician contracted with a group of families to provide care for a regular payment (Abbott 1931).

Health care arrangements in New France were essentially unchanged by the English conquest; most inhabitants chose to remain under the English, who simply replaced French salaries for necessary service providers with British ones. English-speaking physicians arrived with both English and American settlers, and essentially parallel health care arrangements were established for the French and English populations. The first English public hospital was established in Montreal in 1819 through the efforts of the Female Benevolent Society and charitable appeals. By 1823, the medical officers of that institution not only were founding a medical school but were seeking control over medical licensure in the colony on the basis of their supposedly superior British medical educations. This caused resentment among the French-educated doctors, sparking a long conflict between the two medical groups (Abbott 1931).

English Canada was therefore settled much later than French Canada; the Hudson's Bay Company, founded in 1670, had conducted much of the initial exploration of central and western Canada, establishing strategically placed forts and trading posts but resisting settlement. Soldiers, administrators, and their physicians followed the English conquest of 1759, as did British settlers and 35,000 American loyalists in the 1770s; New France (present-day Quebec) became Lower Canada, and present-day Ontario became Upper Canada (McInnis 1959). There was a great deal of farmable land in Upper Canada; land was also granted in 1811 in the Red River area, to the west of Upper Canada, for an agricultural colony there (Mitchell 1954). As a result, the English Canadian population became dispersed over great distances. Most health matters in the rural areas were necessarily handled by individuals or their families. However, colonists in the larger towns, as in French Canada, expected to be treated in their own homes by private physicians, surgeons, apothecaries, or midwives (Shortt 1983–84).

Early Health Care Institutions

As the colonies matured, the population aged as well, and proportionately more colonists who had neither families nor resources to pay for care developed disabilities or chronic illnesses. Under British law, responsibility for these sick poor and aged fell to the municipalities. With municipal governments frequently nonexistent or weak, however, institutions had to be adapted to local conditions. Hospitals for the poor were therefore often organized as charities by groups of relatively prosperous local citizens; where no such groups existed, little assistance was available (Taylor 1978).

One early exception to this pattern was Nova Scotia, where a 1750 parliamentary grant provided funds for both a local hospital to treat soldiers and "miscreants" and salaries for a few surgeons and midwives to attend "sober industrious" indigents at home. This assistance was apparently conceived of as temporary, however; by 1764, the British government had phased out all its assistance except for the hospital (Mackay 1981). Colonial governments were reluctant to subsidize care but found themselves increasingly pressured to do so. By the 1820s, the government of Upper Canada was subsidizing the establishment of charity hospitals there (Godfrey 1979). By confederation in 1867, both Upper and Lower Canada were providing substantial shares of the funding of their privately owned, nonprofit hospitals (Charles and Badgley 1997:3–4). In 1874, the Charity Aid Act authorized provincial subsidies of 20 cents per patient per day for hospital care; by 1882, 12 hospitals were receiving funds under this act. Only in 1912 was municipal responsibility written into law in Ontario, with sufficient provincial grants provided to supplement hospital donations and patient fees (Godfrey 1979:174–85).

By 1891, some parts of Canada had developed fraternal worker organizations that contracted with physicians to provide care for members on either a capitation (per-patient) or fee-for-service basis. Also, some employers at about this time began to insure their employees for both medical and hospital care (Andrews 1981). The state of medical science had improved enough by the 1890s that the technology available in hospitals offered advantages over home care, and some physicians began to seek access to hospital beds for their private patients. Hospitals, finding donations increasingly insufficient to their needs, desired the income from paying customers; they therefore responded by making concessions to physicians with private patients, increasing those doctors' institutional authority, and creating special rooms or wards for private patients. The stigma attached to charity hospitals, therefore, gradually became attached to public ward care only. By 1921, over 70 percent of one major hospital's funding came from patient fees, and physicians' authority was firmly established in hospitals across Canada (Shortt 1983–84).

By the end of the nineteenth century, governments in all the provinces were involved in the provision of public health services, including some "relief" services for the poor (Gray 1991:26–7). However, many Canadian municipalities remained weak and often only marginally able to fulfill their welfare responsibilities. Well into the twentieth century, the distances involved made private physician care frequently unavailable, even for patients with the resources to pay for care, and public hospital care in many areas remained stigmatized as charity (Taylor 1978; Young 1992:91).

Confederation and Societal Change

Upper and Lower Canada were joined by the British government in 1841 into the colony of Canada, which was gradually granted some rights of self-government. Conflict between East (Quebec) and West (Ontario) Canada, however, resulted in frequent governmental deadlock and precipitated efforts to find some more satisfactory political arrangement. Aggressive American expansion was also a concern. Confederation was therefore discussed, and in 1864, a delegation was sent to Prince Edward Island to invite participation of the Maritime colonies in such a federation. Britain encouraged this development, as it meant turning the defense of the North American colonies, and the building of an expensive intercolonial railway, over to the colonists. On July 1, 1867, the British North America Act of the British Parliament created the Dominion of Canada with four provinces: Ontario, Quebec, Nova Scotia, and New Brunswick. Prince

Edward Island did not join the Dominion until 1873, and Newfoundland remained separate until 1949 (McInnis 1959:287–99, 315, 541).

The western provinces developed to some extent from the west coast eastward, in reaction to gold rushes on the coast and aggressive American settlement and expansion. Some features of the land, as well as the climate, made communication and transportation in these Northwest Territories easier with American settlements to the south than with Canadian settlements to the east. Concerned by this, English loyalists organized Vancouver Island as a colony in 1849 and British Columbia in 1858. These two colonies united in 1866 but were not involved in the confederation negotiations that founded the Dominion of Canada. British Columbia officially joined the Dominion in 1871, the same year as Manitoba, created from the Red River colony west of Ontario (McInnis 1959:270–71, 312–15; Mitchell 1954). The remaining two provinces, Alberta and Saskatchewan, were created from the Northwest Territories between British Columbia and Manitoba in 1905 (Neatby 1981).

The political, social, and economic development of Canada, then, varied a great deal from province to province and lagged in several of the western and Maritime provinces as compared to the more central ones. Although the federal Canadian government assisted in settling and developing these provinces, they remained behind for many years in their ability to offer citizens a comfortable life, and to some extent still do. Some idea of the development differential may be obtained from the dates of the founding of provincial public health boards or departments, which required sufficient population, social organization, and resources to bring health issues forward for public action. The Ontario Board of Health was created in 1882 and Quebec's Bureau in 1887. British Columbia, Nova Scotia, and Manitoba took action in 1892 and 1893. Alberta created a department in 1907, as did Saskatchewan in 1909; finally, New Brunswick acted in 1918 and the Dominion itself in 1919 (Heagerty 1928, vol. 1, 337–83).

Political Institutions

Political institutions in the colonies were modeled on those of Britain. While French Canada remained under France, it had been ruled autocratically. Under British rule, the colonists tended to assert their right to some modicum of self-rule as soon as their population and institutional development allowed; colonial parliaments remained, however, in an advisory capacity to the governor generals of the colonies, who answered to British governments (McInnis 1959:63–75, 125–68).

Under the 1867 British North America Act (the Canadian constitution), the parliamentary model was assumed, rather than spelled out, as the form of government. Two parliamentary chambers were established. Particular areas were constitutionally reserved to the provinces, and those not spelled out were assigned to the Dominion government. It was the intent of the founders to create a strong central government; the difficulties of the United States to the south were sufficient to convince the colonial representatives of the necessity of such an arrangement (McInnis 1959:291–92). Except for quarantine measures, the area of health was constitutionally reserved for provincial action (Vayda and Deber 1992).

Initially, there were no formal political parties, and ministers of parliament (MPs) were elected on an individual basis. For its first five years, the Canadian government was composed primarily of the men most active in confederation. Factions formed around cabinet ministers and their supporters, which included many legislators elected for the primary purpose of securing patronage for their districts, or ridings. The opposition at that time consisted of MPs who did not approve of the governing group, plus a disgruntled group of anticonfederation Nova Scotians. Over time, stands on issues divided these legislators into two rudimentary ideological camps, and the governing group formed the nucleus of the Conservative Party, which lost power over a scandal in 1872. The first Liberal government held power for the next five years but with little cohesive policy or organization. In 1878, elections were reorganized to facilitate responsible party government, and those two political parties began consolidating their hold on Canadian politics (Van Loon and Whittington 1976:245–46).

Simultaneous commonwealth elections were instituted in eastern Canada but delayed in the west, which was preoccupied with the need for a transcontinental railway. Nonsimultaneous elections made it possible for westerners to deliberately elect MPs from the winning national party, in order to secure commonwealth support for the railroad; however, this strategy also delayed their adoption of Conservative or Liberal Party loyalties. The lack of a two-party tradition in the western provinces became important in 1919, when the first of a series of western-based third parties made significant gains in a provincial election.

The Progressive Party was made up of farmers and a few small businessmen. This group had become disillusioned with the two major parties, which were dominated by eastern urban and big business interests. In a parliamentary system, strict party discipline is required, leaving no route for a minority faction to achieve political representation within a major political party. The farmers therefore began a protest movement and founded a political party of their own. The Progressive Party's anticaucus ideology resulted in a party structure that proved ineffective nationally but popular at the provincial level; the Progressives held power in Alberta and Manitoba for over two decades. By 1933, this party had been replaced in Saskatchewan by the socialist Cooperative Commonwealth Federation (CCF) and, soon after, by the right-wing populist Social Credit Party in Alberta and British Columbia (Van Loon and Whittington 1976:257–66). Both of these parties have held power in several provinces, achieved representation at the federal level, and survive to the present day.

The other major source of third parties in Canada has been Quebec, which was more successfully penetrated by the Liberals than by the Conservative Party. Dissatisfaction with the Conservatives as an alternative provoked the founding of several uniquely French Canadian parties, including the Union Nationale, the social democratic Parti Quebecois, and the Ralliement des Creditistes, a Quebec-based wing of the Social Credit Party. These parties do not always aspire to national representation, as many French-Canadian politicians regard holding power in Quebec as more important than national office (Van Loon and Whittington 1976:261–68; Olsen 2002).

Labor Development

The organization of labor, which was to prove so critical to future NHI developments, began in the Canadian colonies in the 1830s, with local unions of skilled craftsmen in the York (Toronto), Quebec, Montreal, and Hamilton printing trade. These societies generally took a conciliatory approach to management and varied greatly in their ability to protect or improve the wages or working conditions of their members. The scarcity of skilled labor worked in their favor, but dependence upon a few employers, along with the difficulties of communication and travel for wider organization, worked against them. These unions often included mutual insurance arrangements to protect workers from unemployment and provide for the expenses of illness and death. By the 1860s, Canadian craft unions were flourishing in eastern and central Canada for shipbuilders, bakers, and tailors; however, only one union appears to have existed west of Ontario until 1880 (Logan 1948:23–31; Forsey 1985:10–12).

International unionism in Canada began in 1850 with the establishment of a branch of an English society of engineers in Toronto, soon followed by branches in other communities and an English society of carpenters and joiners in 1860. The early 1860s also saw the organization of the first Canadian branch of an American union, the Iron Molders' Union of North America, soon followed by American societies for typographers, cigarmakers, coopers, locomotive engineers, railway conductors, and shoemakers (Logan 1948:29–31). In this early period, the two nations essentially constituted a single labor market. That is, when jobs were scarce at home, craftsmen often sought work across the border, and membership in an international union simplified the process of getting a job there. Furthermore, the American unions tended to be bigger, better funded, and more experienced in industrial conflict (Forsey 1985:12–13).

The first concerted effort in Canada to win a concession for labor as a class appears to have occurred in Ontario in 1871 with the formation of a nine-hour league; at this time, a strong drive for the nine-hour work day was going on in England, while eight-hour leagues and mass meetings were common in the United States. A parade and mass demonstration was held in Toronto in 1872 to protest the refusal of employers to meet with labor representatives on this issue; the following day, the 24 members of the Typographical Union's committee found themselves arrested on charges of seditious conspiracy. However, as Britain had recently legalized trade unions there, the application of the older British sedition laws to Canadian unions met with widespread outrage, and the typographers' union went on strike. Within months, an act of Parliament had legalized unions in Canada, prosecution of the union committee members was dropped, and the strike had won a nine-hour day for Toronto union printers. This early success appears to have helped unite the Canadian labor movement, establish its respectability, and convince it of the importance of legislation and politics in its struggle (Logan 1948:38–43).

By 1880, unskilled workers were also organizing. The Knights of Labor organized across both crafts and industries, while miners, longshoremen, retail clerks, and railway men became organized along industrial lines. By 1902, the Knights of Labor had dwindled in importance, as the strictly industrial unions proved more effective and durable. It was not until the late 1930s and the formation of the American CIO, however, that industrial unionism really flourished in Canada (Forsey 1985:16–17).

Most Canadian labor remained unorganized until the turn of the century, when the American Federation of Labor (AFL) became concerned that Canadian labor would be used to undercut American unions. The AFL aggressively organized Canadian workers, partially funded the Trades and Labor Congress of Canada (TLCC), and by 1902 was able to pack the TLCC's convention, exclude every organization duplicating an AFL union, and effectively reduce the TLCC to an arm of the AFL. A rival, national labor federation was formed by the excluded Canadian unions, while the powerful TLCC became increasingly divided between western radicalism and the conservatism of the dominant eastern unions (Forsey 1985:13–14; Logan 1948).

The formation of these national labor federations in Canada coincided with formation of the Congress of Industrial Organizations (CIO) in the United States, prompting industrial workers in Canada to organize branches of CIO unions and adopt CIO tactics such as the sit-in strike. The AFL, which was still feuding with the CIO in the United States, had the CIO unions expelled from the TLCC in 1939; however, those unions were able to merge with the rival Canadian labor federation to form the Canadian Congress of Labor (CCL) in 1941. While the CCL also suffered at times from American domination, it maintained more political independence and radicalism than the TLCC and succeeded in organizing the mass production industries in Canada. After the 1955 merger of the AFL-CIO in the United States, the TLCC and CCL merged to form the present Canadian Labor Congress (CLC) in 1956. This national labor congress exists presently alongside the Confederation of National Trade Unions (CNTU), a regional Catholic body that began as a group of conservative, religiously dominated French Canadian unions but evolved during the 1940s into a leader of militant unionism in Quebec (Forsey 1985:17–19; Logan 1948). By the late 1950s, in spite of its later start, Canadian labor organization had caught up with American labor organization.

In terms of achieving its political goals, however, Canadian labor had surpassed American labor by the 1950s. Canadian labor, from quite early, had identified laws it needed and demanded action on them from government. It used two methods of achieving these goals, one modeled on American labor tactics and one on British. The American method is to lobby governments and members of legislatures and then reward its friends and punish its enemies at the ballot box. However, this strategy has real limitations in a parliamentary system, where members of political parties are obliged to vote with their leaders, and an adverse vote on a government bill is almost certain to cause a political crisis and bring on a new election. The only effective lobbying in such a system is of a party's leadership, and whole parties must be cultivated as friends or rejected as enemies.

The British method of independent political action by labor had therefore come into increasing use during the 1880s and 1890s by Canadian unions. This method involved nominating labor candidates for Parliament with no party affiliation; these independent candidates were occasionally elected, but without a party, they proved ineffective in Parliament. A Canadian labor party was founded in 1906 and again in 1917, both times without enough success at the polls to survive. In 1943, the industrially oriented Canadian Congress of Labor formally endorsed the western farm-based Cooperative Commonwealth Federation (CCF) as the "political arm of labour"; this merger enjoyed more support and success in some provinces than others, however, and was never endorsed by the craft-oriented TLCC (Forsey 1985).

The CCF became the official opposition party in British Columbia and Saskatchewan in 1933 and 1934, respectively; by the mid-40s, a CCF government had been formed in Saskatchewan. The CCF also enjoyed some electoral success in Ontario, forming the official opposition more than once and coming close to election as the government. However, the CCF suffered from both internal and external power struggles. Internally, its founding and individual Socialist members were wary of the "reformist" tendencies of the trades unions and resisted full representation for the unions even when most of the CCF's funds and potential votes came from that group. Externally, the rival Labour-Progressive Party (LPP), representing Communist-dominated trade unions during the early 1940s, competed with the CCF for union support through an alliance with the Liberal Party and a "Win the War First" policy. Even after the end of World War II, with the resurgence of union activism and demise of the LPP, the CCF was unable to achieve more than third-party status in Parliament. A prolonged struggle between pro-CCF and anti-CCF leaders in the union movement, plus the merger of the TLCC and CCL, were necessary before Canada's unions aligned themselves with the CCF nationwide (Horowitz 1968).

In 1961, the Canadian Labour Congress and the CCF, after consultation with major farming organizations, founded the New Democratic Party (NDP), which has served as the political voice of Canadian labor since that time. Through the legacy of the CCF, which primarily represented western farmers and "prairie populism" (MacPherson 1979; Lipset 1950), the NDP has retained a broad slice of the rural working class as well as organized labor. However, as the New Democratic Party's structure increased both the formal links and the influence of the unions in the party over those in the CCF, it resolved the struggle within the CCF in favor of the unions, losing some of its socialist farm support in the process (Horowitz 1968). The NDP has enjoyed steadier electoral support than the CCF; however, it has not surpassed the CCF's record of national third-party status combined with success in several provinces.

CANADIAN HEALTH CARE REFORM INITIATIVES

The political struggle for universal access to health care for Canadian citizens began at the provincial level, just after the turn of the century, when some western governments, breaking with the traditions of the more densely populated and privatized east, became involved in the regular provision of medical and hospital care to citizens. These initiatives emerged from the strong rural cooperative movement that appeared in the prairie provinces by the end of the nineteenth century and gained momentum during the depression of the 1930s (McPherson 1979). The Cooperative Commonwealth Federation party was founded as a part of this movement in 1932 (Lipset 1950).

Saskatchewan passed legislation in 1909 enabling municipalities to provide hospital facilities and services. The same province introduced a municipal doctor scheme in 1914, enabling municipalities to contract with doctors to provide medical services to citizens for an annual retainer; this plan later spread to Alberta and Manitoba as well. In 1916, Saskatchewan legislation allowed municipalities to band together in Union Hospital Districts to form a tax base sufficient to construct and support a rural hospital; by 1944, 23 such districts and hospitals had been created (Ostry 1994; Gray 1991:27–28). Building on this legacy, the CCF proposed extensive government intervention in health care in 1933, declaring that health services should be as freely available as educational services and not a matter of private enterprise (Gray 1991:26–28).

In the western provinces, therefore, the governmental provision of health care services or insurance was a recurring theme well before World War II and widely regarded as a simple extension of an already active government role. Health insurance became a political issue in British Columbia in 1919 and in Alberta by the late 1920s; a select committee in Manitoba recommended a mixed program of direct government services and insurance for that province in 1931. As a result of such initiatives, wide public debate had taken place in the western provinces and strong public support for government action existed, well before any provincial health insurance schemes were actually implemented (Gray 1991:28–29).

A government role in health care grew more slowly in the rest of Canada. In 1919, the Liberal Party included a resolution in its platform for governmental insurance against unemployment, sickness, and old age (Bothwell 1977:191). After its election, however, the Liberal government failed to introduce legislation to implement any such programs until 1927 and then only to provide half the funding for provincial old age pensions on a limited, means-tested basis. This was the beginning of Mackenzie King's long tenure as prime minister, which continued through the Second World War (Pickersgill 1977).

The Liberal "promise" was not forgotten, however, and was periodically raised in the House of Commons. A House Select Committee heard testimony on health insurance in 1928 but reported to the House the next year that, in the government's opinion, constitutional jurisdiction over social policy lay exclusively with the provinces (Bothwell 1977:191–92).

During the Depression of the 1930s, declining revenues and the increased need for assistance strained many cities and towns to the point of bankruptcy. With food, clothing, and shelter straining relief budgets, medical care often became unaffordable. Medical association officers lobbied the provincial and commonwealth governments for assistance in providing care; the Dominion government refused, however, on the basis that such matters were "strictly the business of the provinces" (Taylor 1978:4–5). In 1935, Ontario established a fund and an agreement with organized medicine to subsidize medical services for the poor. In the same year, Newfoundland began to provide an extensive range of health services outside its cities through its Cottage Hospital and Medical Care plan. In the other eastern and central provinces, health services remained "a private matter" (Gray 1991:27).

There was no equivalent to Roosevelt's New Deal in Depression-era Canada, and no aggressive commonwealth level effort by either major party to create one. The lack of such a response to the many crises of the Depression helped to build support for the CCF and Canadian socialism (Maioni 1998:53).

The First Federal Health Care Proposal

Social policy became a prominent national issue in Canada during the Second World War. The legacy of the Depression, added to the sacrifices made in the war effort, resulted in a widespread desire to end want, risk, and minimal, begrudging assistance programs. The wartime Liberal government began to plan for a more prosperous postwar period, including full employment and financial protection from unemployment, disability, old age, and sickness (Taylor 1978:2–3). The King government succeeded in getting a constitutional amendment through in 1941 to allow a commonwealth system of unemployment insurance; in 1944, family allowance legislation was passed (Pickersgill 1977:28).

The Liberal government, however, was divided about how much the nation could afford in the way of social programs. While it debated, growing support for the CCF party in the western provinces increasingly pushed health policy into commonwealth politics. The Rowell-Sirois Royal Commission on Dominion-Provincial Relations, appointed in 1937, had added impetus by studying the problem and predicting chaotic results for business if each province acted independently on health insurance. Under the sponsorship of an activist Minister for Pensions and Health, a national health insurance proposal was finally constructed and hearings held; the positions of many organized labor, business, medicine, and other interest groups on NHI appear to have formed during this process. Due to financial and constitutional questions, action on the proposal was delayed until 1945, when it was incorporated into the government's comprehensive 1945 legislative proposals (Gray 1991:30–33; Taylor 1978:7, 16; Maioni 1998:66–73).

These were the famous 1945 Green Book Proposals, embodying the Liberal Party's postwar economic and social policies. Each, like the health insurance proposal, had moved from construction in a governmental ministry to interdepartmental committee consideration and then to a Cabinet committee for final decisions and action. Most, like the health proposal, involved constitutional matters between the provinces and the commonwealth; for that reason, the proposals were presented as a group in the 1945 Dominion-Provincial Conference for negotiation with the provincial governments. Eventually, the health proposal, constructed around a model provincial health insurance bill, was abandoned in favor of a more favorably received "health grants" proposal that would share provincial health costs without requiring specific provincial action on health insurance (Maioni 1998:74–78; Taylor 1978:4, 45; Martin 1977:37–38; Bothwell 1977).

With the Green Book Proposals, the government proposed a radical shift in social provision and tax-sharing arrangements between the commonwealth and provincial governments. First, it proposed that the Dominion assume complete financial responsibility for unemployment assistance and old age pensions. Second, it proposed a transfer of tax fields, wherein the provincial governments would grant the dominion government exclusive access to certain major sources of revenue, and the dominion government would give the provinces exclusive access to other, less lucrative tax fields. Third, it offered to share commonwealth revenues with the provinces in such a way as to stabilize their sources of funding and to make possible a minimum, adequate standard of services in all the provinces. In the health field, this was to take the form of federal health grants to the provinces on a per capita basis, to approximate 60 percent of total costs (Taylor 1978:51–55).

Due largely to the objections of the premiers of Ontario and Quebec to the loss of particular taxes, the 1945–46 dominion-provincial conferences ended with no agreement on the Green Book Proposals. The only health initiative passed at that time was the provision of health grants to help the provinces expand and improve their health care facilities. Considering the central concern with economic policy at that time, it is notable that health policy even was included in the 1945 proposals, much less that they came close to being accepted (Taylor 1978:55; Gray 1991:33). Two important legacies from the 1945 proposals endured to shape future health policy. First, much necessary national research, policy exploration, and public education was accomplished. Second, the health grants created a precedent for a federal role in health care provision and expanded health care facilities nationwide, removing important impediments to the eventual introduction of NHI.

NHI was not taken up again at the commonwealth level until 1955; in the interval, however, several of the western provinces developed and implemented health insurance programs of their own. The first such program was in Saskatchewan. A CCF government, elected there in 1944, immediately began planning and implementing health programs in spite of provincial financial problems and physician opposition. A province-wide hospital insurance plan was passed with minimal controversy in March 1946. Medical service provisions, however, were effectively blocked in all but two regions of the province by medical opposition. In the Swift

Current region of Saskatchewan, a full system of hospital and fee-for-service medical insurance was introduced which later became a prototype for the national program. The negotiated replacement of salaried medical practice with fee-for-service provisions in this program therefore constituted an important victory for organized medicine. The implementation of Saskatchewan's program was made easier by its history of municipal doctor and hospital plans; the Saskatchewan Association of Rural Municipalities both urged the provincial government to adopt such a program and volunteered its members' services to collect the necessary personal taxes (Gray 1991:34–35; Taylor 1990:67–75, 97–98).

British Columbia passed legislation similar to the Saskatchewan Hospitals Service Plan in 1948 but experienced many more problems in its implementation. British Columbia had a large proportion of its population in unorganized parts of the province and had relatively few subscribers to Blue Cross hospitalization insurance, so there was no efficient way to enroll residents or to collect individual premiums. Furthermore, provincial officials underestimated the difficulty of this problem, as well as the lead time necessary to plan and set up the necessary program administration. The resulting confusion and frustration were exacerbated by rising hospital, patient, and program costs. A formal investigation, followed by several resignations, culminated in the defeat of the government in the 1952 elections. Under a new government, changes in the program made it voluntary and then changed the financing to a retail sales tax. Although British Columbia's hospital insurance system was working well by 1954, it long served as an object lesson to other Canadian governments of what to avoid in implementing such a program (Taylor 1990:76–78).

Newfoundland joined the Dominion of Canada in 1949 with an already established cottage hospital system for residents outside its cities. These provincially owned hospitals and salaried physicians were estimated to serve approximately 47 percent of the province's population at the time. Then, with programs in place in the provinces on either side of it, the government of Alberta decided to build in 1950 on its hospitalization programs for maternity, polio, and social assistance recipients. Starting with few municipal plans in place, Alberta adopted a limited scheme subsidizing municipal hospital programs, with plans to expand the scheme in the future. The program did not solve the hospital deficit problem in Alberta; municipalities and religious and other hospital-owning entities still found themselves in financial straits. By 1954, Alberta's program was estimated to cover 75 percent of the population, but only 39 percent of hospital revenues (Taylor 1990:78–80).

These provincial programs changed the federal-provincial dynamic surrounding the public health insurance question. By 1953 the Dominion government, under a more conservative Liberal prime minister, had rejected further federal health insurance initiatives, putting "the ball in the provinces' court." With only three small and one midsized province calling for federal action, the prime minister judged provincial support for a national program to be inadequate; action from one of the large provinces, Ontario or Quebec, would be necessary to move things forward. However, the CCF party whip made a point of embarrassing the government by mentioning its unfulfilled promises and the success of Saskatchewan's hospital insurance program at every opportunity, and public pressure mounted (Taylor 1978:108, 206; Maioni 1998:101).

National Hospital Insurance

By 1954, Ontario's Progressive Conservative government was under pressure to find solutions to a provincial shortage of hospital beds, chronic hospital operating deficits, inadequate private insurance coverage for certain groups, and care access problems among the uninsured. The Ontario Premier, Mr. Frost, was interested in solving these problems; however, he was also interested in seeing an integrated national plan put in place, reducing provincial health care as an issue for his provincial Liberal and CCF opposition, and putting the onus back onto the federal Liberal government for any lack of action. He therefore commissioned research on the Ontario health services situation and publicly raised the issue of a national health insurance program, to the embarrassment of the prime minister, at the 1955 federal provincial conference (Taylor 1978:105–18).

This was followed by two years of political negotiation and bluff between the federal Liberal government and the Progressive Conservative government of Ontario. Prime Minister St. Laurent wanted Ontario to commit itself to a universal provincial hospital insurance program before the Dominion took action; but Premier Frost wanted a federal scheme to integrate and partially fund the provincial programs, while retaining his ability to implement a program for Ontario in stages, with few federal conditions. In the end, after countless studies, meetings, letters, announcements, ultimatums, and compromises, both got their wishes. Enabling legislation was passed in Ontario in March 1956 and March 1957; federal legislation followed in April 1957 (Taylor 1978:124–59). The pressure for action on the federal government came not only from Ontario, however, but also from other provinces, members of the Cabinet, the CCF and Progressive Conservative opposition parties, the public, and the press. In the end, the Liberal government's need to mute criticism in the face of an impending federal election moved the issue forward. Concessions from the federal government led to concessions from the Ontario government, and the Hospital Insurance and Diagnostic Services Act was introduced and passed unanimously in both houses of Parliament. Saskatchewan, Alberta, British Columbia, Manitoba, and Newfoundland's hospital insurance programs began receiving federal subsidies on July 1, 1958. Programs in Ontario, Nova Scotia, New Brunswick, and Prince Edward Island followed in 1959, and Quebec finally joined the hospital insurance scheme in 1961 (Gray 1991:36–37; Taylor 1978:161–234).

Saskatchewan's Medical Insurance Program

The federal hospital insurance program triggered the introduction of a pioneering provincial medical insurance program, again in Saskatchewan. The political struggle over this program, and its outcomes, had lasting effects across Canada, so I will discuss it in some detail.

Federal cost sharing for the Saskatchewan hospital insurance program made it possible for that province's CCF government to budget the last, unfulfilled piece of its 1944 program: universal medical insurance. By 1959, however, Saskatchewan probably represented the toughest province in which to implement such a program. Organized medicine was unusually strong there due to a unique institutional arrangement, in which the provincial medical association, the College of Physicians and Surgeons, served as the legal body responsible for licensing doctors. Membership in this association was compulsory for physician licensure, providing it with more members and funds than was usual for such an association, along with unusual power over physicians who might otherwise dissent from its political stances. This body constituted, in essence, a private government in the field of health. In addition, physician opposition to governmental medical insurance was unusually strong in Saskatchewan, due to the emigration of a number of British doctors to that province after the introduction in Britain of the National Health Service. Ironically, this influx had been encouraged by increased opportunities in Saskatchewan for private medical practice after the introduction of the provincial hospital insurance program (Taylor 1978:264–66).

The college and the Canadian Medical Association (CMA) strongly opposed, and had effectively organized the medical profession against, any government programs that would reduce the profession's economic and clinical autonomy. Physicians had begun encouraging the development of private medical insurance in the 1930s, in the hope of making any public scheme unnecessary; two physician-controlled voluntary insurance programs now dominated medical insurance in Saskatchewan. A commercial health insurance sector also had developed across Canada, which now joined the doctors and the Chamber of Commerce in opposing public provincial medical insurance. However, it was the college's opposition that presented real obstacles for the program (Gray 1991; Taylor 1978).

In spite of college-induced delays and refusals to participate in the planning process, the Saskatchewan Medical Care Insurance Act was passed by the CCF government in 1961; under pressure of a pending 1964 provincial election, the CCF had decided that it could not wait any longer to begin to fulfill such an important part of its platform. However, implementation required consultation and agreements with the representatives of the medical profession. The college hardened its position in opposition, refusing to name delegates to the governing commission, forcing further delays and concessions from the government. However, the college made no substantive concessions in return, and no agreement was in place when the much-delayed startup date finally arrived. The profession's bid for popular support received a boost when the June 18, 1962, federal election turned against the CCF in Saskatchewan. However, since provincial and federal elections are held separately in Canada, the provincial government was not affected (Taylor 1978:239–96).

On July 1, 1962, when the new insurance program was to begin, most of the province's physicians went on strike, withdrawing all but emergency services at a few regional centers. The provincial government had already begun recruiting doctors from outside the province, but many areas were without services, and one child died as a result. Keep Our Doctors (KOD) committees of frightened citizens, backed by the Liberal Party, the American Medical Association, and "a large part of the business and professional power elite of the province" (Badgeley and Wolfe 1967:78), held meetings and rallies all over Saskatchewan in support of the doctors. Virulent anticommunist rhetoric was used to attack the government and its program. On the opposite side, Saskatchewan Citizens for Medicare actively campaigned against the strike, while several communities organized community clinics that planned to recruit doctors on a salaried basis. Most newspapers in Saskatchewan attacked the provincial government's position, while the press outside the province generally expressed more disapproval of the doctors. However, local perceptions began to change when a widely advertised KOD rally on July 11, in front of the Parliament buildings in Regina, failed to draw the large crowd expected. Gradually, public opinion turned against the doctors. Informal negotiations were begun, a prominent British physician was brought in to mediate, and after further governmental concessions, the doctors returned to work. The strike had lasted 23 days (Badgley and Wolfe 1967; Taylor 1990:106–30).

Although Saskatchewan's CCF government won its program, the cost was high; it lost control of the government in the next election, due largely to the enemies it had made in the 1962 struggle. However, the new Liberal government did not terminate the provincial medical insurance program as its opponents had hoped, nor did it change the program to preserve the voluntary insurance programs. Furthermore, the former CCF regained control of the Saskatchewan government in 1971 as the New Democratic Party (NDP), so its political fortunes were not dimmed for long by the 1962 controversy. In addition, the Saskatchewan program's success moved medical insurance forward on the agendas of three other provinces (Taylor 1978:327–30). Indeed, the NDP still appears to be held in some affection by the people of Canada as the initiator of Medicare; to that extent, the struggle to implement the Saskatchewan program may have permanently benefitted Canada's social democratic party.

The public medical insurance program in Saskatchewan was the first such program to be instituted and the first successful confrontation of organized medicine by government in North America. The issues confronted are important to explore, because they were representative of those encountered later in Canadian struggles and because the outcome in Saskatchewan forever changed what had become accepted as the limits of such programs in that nation.

The issues in the Saskatchewan struggle centered on financial and administrative control of the health field. The medical profession considered itself the only source of legitimate governance for any health-related program, but the provincial government considered placing public funds under private administration inconsistent with responsible government. A second issue was a role for the physician-sponsored voluntary insurance programs, which the college attempted to have subsidized and institutionalized as the collector of premiums, insuring body, and dispenser of funds for the province. Preservation of these programs was regarded by the college as nonnegotiable, because they represented the profession's only hope of eventually replacing government insurance and recovering its control of the field. A third issue was control of medical fee levels; the college considered this a professional prerogative, but the government regarded control of medical fee inflation as basic to protecting citizens from the costs of medical care and a reasonable requirement of professional responsibility. A fourth issue concerned the development of regional medical districts; the college opposed this as interfering with professional freedom, since most specialists preferred to practice in the larger cities, but the government wanted a more rational arrangement of services in the largely rural province. Finally, the college maintained that a compulsory universal medical insurance program constituted civil conscription of doctors and was inconsistent with democracy and quality medical care; the government responded that a democratic society ought to be able to organize its medical services for the benefit of its people and that principles of good government were quite consistent with quality care, if not with all professional preferences (Taylor 1978).

In the end, the College of Physicians and Surgeons had to concede governance of the health field to the province; in return, they won a place for voluntary insurance as a program option and the option for physicians to bill their patients instead of the insurance commission, with no check on overall fee inflation. In addition, the government was forced to abandon its plans for regional health districts and had to provide physicians with a number of options that diminished government control over the medical field. In spite of dire predictions, after an initial loss of physicians, the province attracted more doctors than ever before, and physician incomes were the highest in the nation by 1963. By 1970, the program was popular enough with physicians that over 50 percent of Saskatchewan doctors were directly billing the health commission, and the proportion utilizing the voluntary insurance plans was steadily diminishing, increasing the program's ability to control medical inflation (Taylor 1978, 1990).

Canada's federal system thus facilitated the beginning of national health insurance in Canada (Gray 1991:48). Introduction of the system at the provincial level, in Saskatchewan, allowed it to be tested in spite of the opposition of the medical profession; a doctor's strike might well have been impossible to withstand politically either nationally or in any other province, but strong support for the CCF and social democratic policies in Saskatchewan sustained the provincial government through the volatile confrontation. By the time NHI was proposed at the federal level, it had proven both workable and popular in Saskatchewan. This became an important factor in the findings of the Royal Commission on Health Services, which was, ironically, requested by the Canadian Medical Association and appointed by a Progressive Conservative government in the early 1960s. After extensive research and hearings across Canada, which revealed the divisions on this issue between labor and farm groups and medical, insurance and business interests, the Royal Commission presented its recommendations. Those findings included a proposal for programs such as Saskatchewan's in all the provinces (Gray 1991:41–42:Taylor 1990; Maioni 1998:124).

National Medical Insurance

After a significant transformation in the direction of championing social reform, a Liberal Party government was elected in 1963, but with an insufficient majority to rule (Maioni 1998:126–8). With support and pressure from the NDP, and the added impetus of the prestigious Royal Commission's report, the government decided to proceed with national medical insurance. The form of this legislation had to be carefully considered, since the Canadian Medical Association, insurance industry, and at least one provincial government vehemently opposed any plan that replaced voluntary insurance plans with a public scheme. These opponents argued that the government's place in the provision of health insurance was solely to subsidize insurance for the poor. Their arguments had prevailed in the form of provincial medical insurance passed in Alberta in 1963 and were prevailing in the form of legislation on its way to passage in British Columbia (1965) and Ontario (1966) (Taylor 1978:338–41).

However, the Royal Commission's findings strongly recommended against any national scheme that was not both universal and uniform in benefits. In the words of the commission's report, "the number of individuals who would require subsidy to meet total health services is so large that no government could impose the means test procedure on so many citizens, or would be justified in establishing a system requiring so much unnecessary administration" (Hall Report 1964). As Malcolm Taylor interprets the commission's work, these findings posited means testing as inherently undemocratic as well as administratively inefficient; they "used a stigma to beat a dogma," that is, the CMA's doctrine of "individual freedom and the free enterprise system." Furthermore, the commission defended the idea of a compulsory system; as long as the decision was made by a democratically elected legislature, and observed certain limits, the commission expressed confidence that Canadian democratic ideals could not only be protected in such a scheme, but "more fully realized" (Taylor 1990:138–39; Hall Report 1964).

The form of a federal initiative was further complicated by the opposition that had developed in Quebec and Ontario to federal provisions controlling the form of provincial programs in exchange for funding. In order to obtain provincial support, the prime minister decided that federal requirements must be kept to a minimum. The standards or principles decided on, however, favored a Saskatchewan-type program rather than the CMA-favored format prevailing in Alberta, British Columbia, and Ontario. This decision was based primarily on evidence from Australia and Alberta that means-tested programs, based on voluntary insurance and government subsidy or coverage of the poor, did not achieve universal coverage. It was decided that commonwealth funding would be offered for provincial health care programs that were comprehensive, universal, portable, and publicly administered; later, accessibility (i.e., affordable at the point of care) was added (Gray 1991:42–43, 222; Taylor 1978:364–65).

Intensive negotiations with the provinces were necessary to reach realistic compromises on dominion and provincial rights and responsibilities, as well as funding and administrative structures. The result was a proposal that appeared to capitulate to the provinces but gave the commonwealth government a strong role in the health care field; this was put to the provinces at the July 19, 1965, federal-provincial conference (Ruggie 1996:97–100).

The response from the provinces was mixed, with no outright opposition expressed at the conference. However, opposition began to mount in several provinces as the meaning of the federal "principles" became clearer. At the same time, a federal election was coming up, and the ensuing campaign both focused attention on the issue and provided plenty of opportunity for the proposal's opponents to publicize their objections. The Liberal government was returned to power with a marginal gain in Parliament; its medical insurance proposal appeared to be neither rejected nor strongly endorsed by this election result (Taylor 1978:366–67).

A different threat to "Medicare" had been forming in the years since the Pearson government's first election—that of financial constraints. A downturn in the Canadian economy had worsened the budget picture, resulting in opposition within the Cabinet to the expensive new medical insurance program. Traditionally, the minister of finance was the brake on costly new programs, a pattern that had not been present in the previous Pearson government only because the minister of finance for those years, Walter Gordon, was a longtime supporter of NHI. With a new minister of finance and increasingly negative financial projections, both the second reading of the bill and the government's projected date to implement the new program were delayed. However, strong pressure from the NDP and support from the Liberal caucus, especially that of several Cabinet members, kept the legislation from being further delayed or abandoned. The bill successfully passed its third reading in the House on December 8, 1966, and was passed by the Senate on December 16. Even then, the opposition of the minister of finance continued to threaten the program's implementation; a final decision at an emergency Cabinet meeting in November 1967 was necessary to overrule his objections (Taylor 1978:360–74; Maioni 1998:133–35).

Opposition then was concentrated in the provinces to block the implementation of the new national program; Alberta, Ontario, and Quebec fought hard for concessions from the commonwealth to accommodate programs incorporating voluntary insurance and other physician preferences. By January 1971, however, all 10 provinces had joined the national scheme, and Medicare was a national reality. Quebec was the only province to experience real confrontation with its physicians in this process; provisions in Quebec's bill made concessions to organized medicine that antagonized the teachers', farmers', and labor unions, and the association of medical specialists (FMSQ) demanded still more concessions. Under threat of a specialists' strike, the government offered some minor concessions, which were not accepted by the FMSQ. By October 1970, 75 percent of the specialists had left the province. At this point, a political crisis intervened with the kidnapping of a British diplomat and the kidnapping and murder of the minister of labor by the Front de Liberation du Quebec (FLQ). In the emergency that followed, the specialists were ordered to return to work, and after an initial refusal, they complied (Gray 1991:44–47).

Notably, the health care provision system created by these events diverged from the rest of Canada's welfare state, chiefly through its universality. In the years to follow, Medicare's extreme popularity would allow it to diverge somewhat in other ways but without provoking similar changes in approach to other Canadian programs (Banting 1997; Olsen 1994).

Although organized medicine lost the national medical insurance battle, it and its allies had managed to produce a good deal of delay and controversy, increasing the political costs of passage and implementation. Furthermore, they succeeded in changing the form of legislation to maintain private, fee-for-service practice, as well as to remove all effective measures for controlling medical costs. For the next two decades, physicians continued to independently establish fees, without regard for the fee schedules determining government insurance payments, and to bill patients directly for the difference. This practice, which came to be known as "extra-billing," became increasingly controversial between 1970 and 1984; as provincial reimbursement fell further behind the costs of medical care, increased numbers of patients found themselves unable to afford their share of the bill. In spite of vocal NDP criticism, Medicare began increasingly to resemble a 2-tier system (Gray 1991:104–23).

Political Consolidation

The compromises built into both health insurance bills soon created new tensions, including rapid inflation in health care costs. Both the commonwealth and provincial governments encountered difficulties in meeting their financial obligations; each had some reason to blame the other for their problems controlling costs, and Medicare's funding mechanisms had to be renegotiated. However, some of the escalating price tag was clearly due to the practice of extra billing; both physicians' incomes and their numbers increased rapidly after 1970 (Ruggie 1996:100–01).

It was not until 1984, with the Canada Health Act, that direct patient billing within Medicare was ended, a step that effectively brought medical costs under provincial authority and under public control. The bill was introduced by the Liberal opposition, presumably in preparation for the 1984 election; however, the Progressive Conservative government gave the bill its support as well, and it was passed unanimously. Under its provisions, federal financial support would only continue to provinces that enforced rate schedules by outlawing extra billing, taking responsibility for meeting all five of the standards specified at the commonwealth level (Gray 1991:124–25).

This change was bitterly opposed by the medical profession and the provinces, which regarded the change as an intrusion into their prerogatives. Medicare was extremely popular with the general public, however, and its strengthening at the federal level proved politically impossible to stop (Evans 1988:173–74; Gray 1991:128–30). Considering the conservative political trends challenging advocates of NHI at that time in Britain, Europe, and the United States, this 1984 move to strengthen NHI in Canada appears even more remarkable.

Since 1984, Canadian Medicare has suffered from a gradual reduction in commonwealth funding and a parallel increase in the provinces' ability to interpret the five federal conditions in divergent ways. As a result, many hospital services have been decreased and more of their costs shifted onto patients, raising questions about both quality of care and accessibility (Olsen 2002:179–81). As of 1997, Banting concluded that equity of access had essentially been preserved (1997:289). By 2002, however, Olsen concluded that a two-tier system was emerging in Canada, which increasingly allows higher income citizens to procure better health care than lower income citizens (2002:179).

THEORETICAL EXPLANATIONS AND CANADIAN HEALTH POLICY

The Liberal Party, an approximate Canadian parallel to the U.S. Democratic Party, sponsored all the federal legislation that created NHI in Canada. However, the socialist New Democratic Party actually pushed NHI onto the policy agenda at both the provincial and federal levels and gets primary credit for it from the Canadian people. For this reason, Canadian NHI yields more class-based features than might be obvious initially.

For instance, NHI was promised by the Liberal Party in 1919 because of its wide popular appeal. However, no action was taken on it for many years by Liberal governments; the reason given was always budget constraints or economic concerns, presumably a matter of business objections. NHI was first included on a Liberal government's platform only after the appearance of a regional socialist party (the CCF/NDP); furthermore, it proposed no NHI legislation until the 1950s, after the CCF had won provincial power and pioneered a universal hospital insurance program. Finally, it was not until 1966, after the provincially based national hospitalization insurance program had proven both workable and highly popular, the NDP had absorbed the high costs of pioneering a provincial medical insurance program, and the NDP had become a national party threatening the Liberal Party's political base, that a commonwealth Liberal government acted to add medical insurance to the program. This fits the pattern of a conservative government passing worker-friendly legislation to prevent the growth of radical political organizations, including a socialist political party.

Political institutions appear to have facilitated the passage of NHI in Canada in several ways. First of all, there are literally no veto points in Canada except the Constitution, as interpreted by the courts, to constrain the commonwealth government. A government with a clear majority in Parliament may pass whatever legislation it decides upon and expects to be held accountable for those decisions at the next election. With no ability to stop legislation either directly or indirectly, the opposition often finds it worthwhile to support particularly popular legislation. Once a Canadian government became committed to designing and introducing NHI legislation, then, this lack of veto points facilitated its passage.

Second, the principle constraint imposed on NHI by the Constitution of Canada is that giving control over the area of health care to the provinces. Federal financial leverage is provided by court interpretations giving the commonwealth dominance over the most lucrative tax fields and by the tendency of the different levels of government to negotiate agreements rather than test the limits of constitutional privilege in the courts. This last tendency may be encouraged by governmental accountability, as voters are not particularly tolerant of legal challenges and delays. Constitutional and parliamentary institutions in Canada, then, facilitate whatever actions the two primary levels of government can agree upon. The main limits on such agreements are incompatibilities in the agendas of the provincial and commonwealth governments and the skill of policy promoters in finding ways to overcome them. Broad class agendas appear to be as facilitated by this arrangement as narrow interest-group agendas.

Third, Canadian institutions and dynamics appear to have facilitated the appearance, growth, and influence of a socialist third party. The combination of regional divisions and parliamentary government has spawned several third parties, and the tension between the commonwealth and provincial levels of government has supported the growth of these parties at the provincial level. That is, when neither major party at the commonwealth level has appeared representative of a province's sentiments, third-party provincial governments have been very effective at putting the province's views on the national agenda. This has happened in

Quebec with Francophile issues, in Saskatchewan with the CCF/NDP and public health insurance, and in British Columbia and Alberta with the Social Credit Party and regional economic issues. Canada's mainstream parties have then moved to incorporate such issues, but only after their developing sufficient national salience to threaten the dominant two-party pattern.

Canada's path to NHI, then, calls attention to its parliamentary system and relative lack of veto points, its effective constitutional division of powers between the commonwealth and provinces, and the survival and growth of a socialist third party. Canada's regional divisions also appear to have contributed to its legacy of federal-provincial negotiations and compromises, as well as to the development of rural socialism and public health insurance in Saskatchewan.

CHAPTER 3

Australia

Australia's national health policy has had a rockier history than that of any other democratic industrialized nation. Australia is the only such nation to have completely dismantled its system of national health insurance, after once instituting it, and then to have reinstated it once again. Similarly, the history of the passage of NHI in Australia has been a rocky one, characterized by very different Labor and non-Labor Party positions on health policy and by repeated refusals of the Australian Medical Association to obey laws it disliked (Gray 1991; Sax 1984).

This history is a direct result of the political polarization of Australian society. The extreme systemic changes are made possible by Australia's parliamentary system, combined with a 1946 constitutional amendment that first gave the commonwealth—and therefore the party in power at the federal level—broad powers in all aspects of health policy. As a result, "every change in government at the federal level since the 1940s has been followed by a major change in health policy" (Gray 1991).

HISTORICAL INFLUENCES AND LEGACIES

Australia's history of government involvement in health care goes back to its colonial period, with hospitals set up by the British government to provide care for transported convicts. The colonial medical service was established with the arrival of the First Fleet at New South Wales in 1788; four naval surgeons and two medical officers were given the task of creating a base from which services could be given. These tents were soon full of scurvy and dysentery patients, and a more permanent hospital was seen to be necessary. The new structure became the General Hospital (Sax 1984:3). This hospital became the prototype for convict hospitals, and later for public hospitals, in Australia.

A network of convict hospitals was established, run by the colonial medical service and serving as bases for itinerant medical services. Separate wards were maintained for troops and prisoners, and no charges were levied for patient care until 1839 (Sax 1984:4). So the first health policy legacy in the Australian colonies was one of direct and free hospital-based health service provision through the British colonial service.

By 1820, the colonial medical service was being supplemented by private medical practitioners and private care facilities for the free settlers and emancipated prisoners, who were expected to provide for their own needs. As in Britain, private medical care was conceptualized as normal, but as in Canada, frontier conditions made that model problematic. Furthermore, even fewer Australian than Canadian colonists could afford private care. Outpatient treatment was first made available to poor free colonists in 1827 at the Sydney Dispensary, run by a charity group. By 1839, a fee schedule shows that some free persons were allowed to use the convict hospitals, either by qualifying as paupers or by paying a fee (Sax 1984:4, 7).

These innovations were responses to the Australian colonies' glaring problem of the time, the desperate neediness of indigent free persons. In England, these persons would have been cared for at home, by relatives, friends, or neighbors; for most colonists, however, those social networks had been disrupted by transportation or emigration. Furthermore, there was no established system of medieval social organization or church administration in the colonies, as there was in Britain. Without preexisting networks of social assistance, there was an obvious need for new sources of care. Government already filled some of those needs; benevolent societies were founded to meet others.

Starting with "outdoor relief" (nonresidential), and progressing to asylums and "indoor relief" (residence-based), benevolent societies used private donations and government subsidies to run homes and hospitals for insane, disabled, aged, and sick free persons. However, because these institutions developed an ugly likeness to English workhouses and were stigmatized as charity, they were avoided by free colonists and did not meet the need for care (Sax 1984:4–7).

Public Hospitals and Friendly Societies

Once the transportation of prisoners stopped in the 1840s, the colonial government began to withdraw from direct services for soldiers and convicts, and the convict hospitals were gradually turned over to benevolent societies to administer as public hospitals for the poor (Sax 1984:4–7). By the mid-1800s, public hospitals were jointly financed by government, charity, and patient fees, while the medical care in those institutions was provided for free by "honorary" (unpaid) physicians with successful private practices. These institutions provided for the hospital needs of those patients neither poor nor able to afford private hospital care; however, there was still no systemic solution to the outpatient medical needs of this group.

One solution to the medical needs of the working poor was created in New South Wales in the 1830s with the first friendly society, a form of workers' mutual aid organization first developed in Europe and legally accepted in England by 1793. These workers' clubs or lodges represented a proud working-class tradition of independence from either charity or government through mutual assistance. Friendly societies protected their members from funeral expenses and the loss of income associated with sickness through funds maintained by small, regular contributions. They also contracted with physicians to provide medical attendance for members and their families who opted to pay an additional regular fee. Doctors initially appreciated this arrangement, as it gave them a regular source of income while they built up more lucrative and prestigious private practices. However, physicians came to resent such contracts by 1909, claiming that the fees offered were too low, that some society members ought to be paying for private care, and that the arrangement was restricting the growth of private practice (Green and Cromwell 1984).

Another new development, in 1857, was the establishment of the first religious hospital in Australia, St. Vincent's Hospital in Sydney. Religious hospitals initially provided hospital care and inpatient medical services for members of their own religious groups. As such hospitals grew, however, they found it increasingly necessary to seek and accept governmental subsidies and were gradually incorporated into the public hospital system. In some religious hospitals, both public and private proprietary wings were maintained (Sax 1984:24).

The status of physicians remained generally low throughout the colonies' first hundred years, based more on social class than on medical effectiveness. Without a recognized body of medical knowledge, treatment was often ineffective or dangerous, and most patients picked their consultant by price rather than education. By 1881, a wide range of registered and unregistered practitioners provided medical care and advice in

Victoria; only 23 percent of those practitioners consisted of registered physicians, whose professional status was just beginning to increase with their competency. Chemists provided 40 percent of medical care, midwives provided 27 percent, and herbalists, "galvanists," and clairvoyants provided 5 percent (Sax 1984:12–13). Over time, the use of unregistered and alternative practitioners decreased with the development of effective medical treatments and training and with the organization of physicians around protecting and controlling the legal practice of medicine.

Societal Change and Federation

Meanwhile, the Australian colonies were undergoing rapid expansion and growth. The original British colony, carved out with convict labor in the 1780s and 90s, had been New South Wales, on the southeast coast of the Australian continent. Exploration and the immigration of free settlers had prompted the colonization of Tasmania in 1825, Western Australia in 1829, and South Australia in 1834. A gold rush brought many new immigrants to all the colonies, especially New South Wales, the southern portion of which became a separate colony (Victoria) in 1851. Queensland, the last colony to be established, broke off from northern New South Wales in 1859, and by 1860, all the colonies except Queensland had experienced population booms. Assisted immigration and cheap land encouraged rapid growth, although economic hardship and periodic droughts had made both controversial by 1858. By 1891, the population of the six colonies was 3 million and growing fast (Shaw 1955).

Economic and political changes followed. Throughout the nineteenth century, the developing economy of the colonies had been agricultural and extractive, with fledgling industries concentrated initially in Sydney, New South Wales. Colonial policy did not encourage manufacturing, as it would compete with British industry. However, population booms created a need for jobs, which were seasonal in agriculture and insufficient elsewhere; economic problems culminated in depressions and labor organization in the 1840s and 1850s. Laws to protect local products from foreign competition were introduced in 1861 and passed in all the colonies by 1875, in spite of British opposition (Shaw 1955:84–146). Between 1860 and 1890, the colonies enjoyed thirty years of relative prosperity, and Australia was advertised abroad as "the worker's paradise" (Butlin, Barnard, and Pincus 1982). However, the 1890s brought drought and more depression, followed by worker agitation, labor organization, and strikes (Sax 1984:31–32).

In response to the sense of economic crisis, colony leaders sought a way to reduce trade barriers between the colonies to increase commerce. Federation, an idea discussed since 1850 and actively promoted by 1890, became the answer. Nationhood was touted as a way to make Australian products more saleable worldwide, especially in Britain. After much controversy and two referendums, the terms of federation were settled. The Commonwealth Constitution Act was passed by the British Parliament, and the Commonwealth of Australia came into existence on January 1, 1901 (Shaw 1955:182–96). Ongoing labor troubles were then temporarily reconciled by a commonwealth agreement called the "New Protection," which improved workers' wages, offered both manufacturers and workers protection from imported competition, and established a system to arbitrate disputes (Sax 1984). The new nation developed several political parties, including both a strong labor party and a number of conservative parties, which were frequently forced to work together as the anti-labor "non-Labor" coalition.

The Constitution gave the commonwealth government specific and limited powers, including the power to establish laws protecting public health; all other health-related powers were reserved to the states. However, as in Canada, the Constitution gave most of the power to raise funds to the commonwealth, a power that would prove crucial to the development of health care policy in Australia.

New and Politicized Health Care Arrangements

The early 1900s were a time of rapid change in health care arrangements for the new nation. In the area of public health, school health services began in 1907, concern over maternal and infant mortality rates prompted a federal maternity grant of 5 pounds per birth in 1912, and the first public baby clinic was opened in 1914. By 1916, organized physicians were seeking to limit school and baby clinic care, in order to protect the demand for private doctors (Sax 1984:18–19).

In private practice, doctors were organizing to force the friendly societies to increase the medical fees paid and to limit both the services included and the patients covered by their contracts. This "Battle of the Clubs" was fought on the physician side with organization and recruitment, coordinated demands, mass resignations from contract practice, and refusals to consult with contracting doctors. The friendly societies responded by finding or importing new contract doctors and by adjusting the contracts when necessary. In 1909, the Australian Medical Association[1] got an income limit accepted for new friendly society members in New South Wales; this was the first real victory for organized medicine in its battle to set the terms of medical practice (Green and Cromwell 1984).

In 1914 the AMA initiated the Common Form of Agreement, a standardized contract stipulating that new friendly society members had to be examined and accepted by lodge physicians and allowing contracting doctors to charge private fees for certain services. In Victoria, doctors were unable to get the Common Form of Agreement accepted until World War I created a physician shortage; in 1918, they resigned en masse from the friendly societies and treated patients on a fee-for-service basis only until the Common Form was accepted. Ironically, this forced many workers into the public care system, as they could no longer afford friendly society medical care. The peak of friendly society membership occurred in 1913; by 1922, their battle with the AMA was over, and the doctors had won (Green and Cromwell 1984; Sax 1984).

During the early years of the century, free hospitalization became a political issue at the state level. The public hospitals had become much more popular as the effectiveness of new medical treatments became clear, but patient fees limited their availability for many citizens. The New South Wales Political Labor League called for universal, free public hospital care in 1908, to be paid for by local taxes. However, upon election in 1910, Labor was unable to put a state program into place because of AMA and hospital board opposition and because it did not have a sufficient parliamentary majority to force the issue (Sax 1984:25).

On the federal level, the 1919 influenza outbreak tested the limits of Commonwealth authority as controversy erupted over quarantine issues, with some states defying the constitutional responsibility given to the commonwealth for public health. One indicator of the limited federal role at that time is that no commonwealth department of health was even established until 1921 (Sax 1984:16).

AUSTRALIAN HEALTH CARE REFORM INITIATIVES

Some welfare state issues became national political concerns in the early 1900s. Old age pensions were established in 1909, and by 1923, a conservative government was considering a national program to provide the "deserving" poor with income during sickness, invalidity, unemployment, and old age. A royal commission was appointed to consider the issue; its report resulted in the National Insurance Bill of 1928, which would have established compulsory income insurance financed by flat rate contributions from both employers and employees. After introducing the legislation, however, the government abandoned it as a burden on industry (Sax 1984:36).

A separate royal commission was appointed in 1925 to consider health issues. It established a pattern in the consideration of national health issues by being made up mostly of medical doctors, probably through the intervention of a physician member of the Cabinet. This commission recommended cooperative national planning and medical research but no hospital or medical insurance programs. No new commonwealth legislation providing for access to medical care was introduced until 1938, at the end of the Depression (Sax 1984:37–39).

The 1938 Non-Labor Bill

The non-Labor coalition's National Health and Pensions Insurance Bill of 1938 proposed cash benefits for sickness, disability, old age, and widowhood, combined with the creation of a general practitioner medical service. It was to be paid for by employer and employee contributions, supplemented by general revenues. It was also to be compulsory and limited to low-income workers, excluding dependents and the self-employed, and would not have covered births and operations (Sax 1984:39).

In spite of its limitations, this bill was remarkable in several ways. It was the first legislative proposal for a medical service put forward by any Australian government. It also was the first and only attempt by a non-Labor commonwealth government to overrule the wishes of organized medicine. By testing the power of organized medicine, it helped to galvanize that profession into a cohesive and politically effective force. Finally, it represents the first occasion on which organized medicine managed, by noncooperation, to reverse health policy legislation at the federal level.

At the time, however, the bill was controversial for other reasons, perhaps related to its development from British advice poorly suited to the Australian context. The Australian Labor Party objected to new, compulsory contributions from low-income employees. Friendly society members feared government coercion and disruption of their group medical arrangements; they agitated to be allowed to collect the contributions and arrange the benefits. Finally, members of the governing non-Labor coalition demanded that small farmers and other self-employed persons be included in the program, extracting promises for expansion even before the bill was passed in July 1938.

The federal council of the AMA, convinced that some insurance scheme was inevitable, negotiated with the government and agreed upon terms for the medical service. However, the refusal of regular AMA members to endorse the agreement forced the AMA council to withdraw its acceptance and twice delayed the government's implementation date because agreement with the doctors could not be reached. By June 1939, the approach of war pushed other priorities to the fore, and the government was forced to postpone the entire scheme indefinitely (Sax 1984:39–42). Organized medicine had refused to cooperate with the law, stymied the elected national government, and gotten away with it.

The solidarity of Australian physicians on the 1938 bill was critical, so it will be explored in some detail. This unity was the result of their earlier struggle with friendly societies, their current struggles with public hospitals, and their awareness of developments abroad. By the 1930s, conflict had become acute between the public hospitals, which had gradually expanded their services to moderate income patients, and physicians, who were generally unwilling to treat such patients in public hospitals at all except where private hospitals were scarce. Organized doctors regarded private medical care as its normal form and saw the expansion of public systems as unfair competition, a threat to the expansion of private practice. The issue had come to a head in Tasmania, where honorary physicians withdrew their services from public hospitals. Organized medicine lost this early battle; the doctors were replaced by salaried staff doctors (Sax 1984:42–43). The lesson of such losses was not lost on the AMA; its drive to control Australian conditions of practice was clearly threatened by any lack of physician unity.

The consequences of such disunity were also seen in developments overseas, particularly in Britain, where a public medical service had replaced private practice for a significant proportion of Britain's physicians. In Britain and most of Europe, medical unity had been much influenced by hospital arrangements, which evolved from a system of provision for the sick poor, who had no private physicians to attend them. In Europe, a class of salaried physicians became established in the hospitals, while in Britain, honorary (unpaid) posts in public hospitals became a prestigious reward for successful private practice. In both, the hospital-affiliated physicians were in the best position to specialize as medical knowledge improved and gradually formed a separate class of practitioners. In these nations, the medical profession became effectively divided into two classes of practitioner, with different interests (Sax 1984:45).

The evolution of medical insurance had further divided these medical practitioners. Voluntary insurance was introduced through friendly societies in continental Europe very early, and in Britain somewhat later, institutionalizing contract arrangements that controlled the practices and limited the incomes of general medical practitioners. The rarer specialists, more in demand by private patients, were not affected. When these nations then began to establish either national medical services or compulsory health insurance, there were few objections from the prestigious specialists, who did not feel threatened. However, the increasing need for specialist services soon brought them under government financing arrangements as well, provoking bitter resentment at the loss of control over their practices and incomes.

Organized physicians in Australia were aware of different hospital and financing arrangements in the United States, which tended to encourage medical unity. Medical emigrants there had been overwhelmingly general practitioners, and arrangements had evolved in which patients were treated by the same physician, on a fee-for-service basis, both inside and outside of the hospital. This arrangement gave both general practitioners and specialists a strong interest in protecting fee-for-service practice, fostering more solidarity among doctors than was common in Europe. This arrangement had become common in the private hospitals of Australia as well, existing alongside the British system of honorary care in public hospitals (Sax 1984).

By 1938, organized physicians in Australia were determined to protect and foster their unity and autonomy through the fee-for-service system and had settled on a way in which to do it, a voluntary system of provider-controlled medical insurance based on the new hospital contribution funds. This private insurance model was created in 1931 by hospitals and physicians in Sydney; it entitled subscribers with limited means to free public hospital care, while more affluent subscribers had their public or private hospital costs reduced or partly reimbursed. However, subscribers became ineligible for public hospital outpatient services and could for the first time be charged by physicians for their care in public hospitals. In effect, affordable hospital care was offered to subscribers in return for stable hospital income and the shifting of moderate income subscribers into private, fee-for-service physician care arrangements. The scheme was successful, spreading through most of the states so that by the mid-1930s, nearly 30 percent of public hospital costs were being met by private insurance, and private services had gained a larger share of the medical market. Efforts failed to get such funds accepted in Queensland and Tasmania, however; in those states, medical appointments in public hospitals were put on a salaried basis instead (Sax 1984:44).

At the beginning of World War II, then, Australian patients tended to use public hospitals and outpatient medical services when available but were increasingly being pushed into more expensive private care through the efforts of organized medicine. The growing middle class, in particular, felt squeezed by its lack of access to publicly funded but means-tested services and was increasingly resentful of that fact.

The strains caused by these problems resulted in widely varied arrangements at the state level, with numerous programs in place both to provide direct care and to underwrite the cost of care given privately. The national Australian government had little ability to coordinate or rationalize these arrangements, as it had no constitutional authority in the health care area (Gray 1991). Although the issue of constitutionality had not been raised as an objection against non-Labor's 1938 bill to insure low-income workers, it became very much an issue when a new Labor government attempted to ensure access to services for all Australians.

The Free Hospital Experiment

In October 1941, a Labor government was elected, led by a prime minister who had previously declared that "national health services should be treated, in principle, in the same way as education. They should be free to all members of the community" (CPD 1938:155, quoted in Sax 1984:49). In office, this policy was clarified as endorsing the continuance of private practice alongside a salaried medical service, free to all persons wishing to use it. The service was to be financed from tax revenues and to be voluntary for both physicians and patients. World War II forced the postponement of action on social policy until November 1942; however, once the immediate threat to the nation had receded, the Chifley government embarked on an ambitious process of planning for postwar reconstruction and a national welfare program, including health services (Sax 1984:50).

The first step in this program was to provide evidence that financing was available for such programs; this need was met by the establishment in 1943 of the National Welfare Fund and the 1945 division of income tax revenues into two streams, one of which went into that fund. The National Welfare Fund also received payroll tax contributions, and all social services were paid out of it, including hospital benefits and income protection during sickness (Sax 1984:50–51). The commonwealth's ability to finance programs was also improved in 1942 by a High Court ruling that the constitution gave the federal level of government a monopoly on income taxation; this cut off a source of revenue for the states and increased commonwealth leverage on state programs requiring significant funding.

An equally important step was altering the Constitution to clearly authorize Labor's program. A general amendment increasing commonwealth power failed in a 1944 referendum, but an amendment expanding the authority of the federal government in social services alone was approved in a 1946 referendum. This act specifically authorized the commonwealth to make laws with respect to "the provision of . . . pharmaceutical, sickness and hospital benefits, medical and dental services (but not so as to authorize any form of civil conscription)" (Sawer 1988:48). The words in parentheses were introduced in an amendment by the non-Labor opposition and accepted by the Chifley government as a concession to organized medicine (Sax 1984:54–55).

The government's attempts to introduce a salaried medical and dental service, however, were stymied by the Australian Medical Association's refusal to cooperate with the planning process. AMA officials agreed that the Commonwealth could finance new medical clinic, but insisted that physicians control such clinics, that medical payments remain on a fee-for-service basis, and that physician fees remain unconstrained by program benefits. The government would not agree to the private control of public clinics or to a program without fee restrictions, and negotiations ceased.

In retaliation, the AMA reversed itself on cooperation with the Labor government's 1944 Pharmaceutical Benefits Act, which required use of an official formulary (list) and prescription form to provide critical medicines to patients free of charge. Even the passage of a second Pharmaceutical Benefits Act and a 1949 amendment making the use of the form mandatory did not resolve the situation; the AMA challenged this legislation as "civil conscription" under the 1946 constitutional amendment, and the High Court ruled in its favor. The partisan nature of this AMA obstruction is shown in the fact that physicians later accepted an identical arrangement under a non-Labor government (Sax 1984:52–55, 61; Butlin et al. 1982).

The Chifley government's program of free public hospitalization was more successful. The Hospital Benefits Act of 1945 authorized agreements with the states, subsidizing state hospital benefit programs with common-wealth funds. Participating states had to create programs providing for universal, free treatment in the public wards of public hospitals and reduc-ing the cost of treatment in the private wards of those hospitals. Although the AMA objected to this legislation as well, no agreement with them was needed, so they were not able to obstruct it. By the end of 1946, the "free hospital experiment" was working smoothly, though by 1949 hospitals were complaining that the increased government support had resulted in a loss of charitable support and that federal subsidies were not meeting costs (Sax 1984:56–57). This policy initiated state dependence on federal health dollars and the need for state governments to build health care costs and inflation into their budgets, placing state governments of both parties at odds with organized medicine over its professional claims and financial demands.

The final 1940s Labor effort in the health field was the National Health Service Act of 1948. Despairing of reaching agreement with the AMA, which refused either to negotiate or to cooperate, the government authorized in this act the provision of medical and dental services, grants for hospital construction and maintenance by the states, the training of health personnel, and the establishment of health centers and clinics. However, the Chifley government did not get to oversee this act's imple-mentation. The AMA joined non-Labor in campaigning against the Labor government, characterizing it as socialist and dangerous (Sax 1984:58–59). The Labor government was overturned in the election of December 1949, just as the long postwar period of prosperity began to be felt in Australia, the United States, and Canada.

The Dissolution of the Free Hospital Experiment

The new, non-Labor government used the legislation passed by the Labor government to institute a voluntary system of medical insurance that accommodated the demands of the medical profession and the concerns of financial conservatives. It also ended the free hospitalization policy in

1952, citing the cost of the policy as a strain on the economy (Gray 1991:91–94). These alterations set the pattern for non-Labor policy for the next fifty years, creating new financial strains for moderate and low-income patients but satisfying many of the health care needs of more affluent workers. Lasting for over two decades, the Menzies government's health care policy subsidized and helped to build up private insurance, private hospitals, and private medical practice in Australia.

There were four parts to this market-oriented policy. The first was pharmaceutical benefits, structured very much as the previous Labor government had proposed but now enjoying the full cooperation of the doctors (Sax 1984:53–55, 60–61).

Another was the new Hospital Benefits Act. This legislation provided more per patient federal grant money to the states for hospital and nursing home care, especially for pensioners and their dependents, who were provided for at a much higher rate than other citizens. States were allowed to begin charging hospital patients using public wards, making them subject once again to means testing. In addition, a policy to encourage voluntary hospital insurance was instituted, which paid extra benefits to patients insured through approved nonprofit organizations. As most insurance funds did not cover preexisting or chronic illnesses, however, many insurees were insufficiently protected by this act, which was amended in 1958, 1962, and 1969. Uninsured patients were also insufficiently protected but received no similar relief (Sax 1984:61–64).

A third part of the Menzies policy was its medical benefits system. Like the hospital act, this legislation provided for cash benefits tied to voluntary medical insurance through registered nonprofit insurance funds. This act incorporated all the demands of the AMA: patients were to pay both their insurers and doctors directly; patients would then be reimbursed for up to 90 percent of their medical costs by their insurer, which would be partly reimbursed by the commonwealth; and insurance benefits would have no limiting effect on physician fees. Both physician-sponsored contribution funds and friendly societies became registered insurance organizations under this policy (Sax 1984:64–65).

The fourth was a pensioner medical service, which put low-income retirees on a different benefit basis than all other citizens and made general practitioner medical services available to them and their dependents, subject to a means test. MDs agreed to be paid from a negotiated fee schedule for this service; the fee schedule and the means test, however, proved to be constant sources of friction, undergoing major renegotiation and change at least five times over the next two decades. Eventually, alleged physician abuse of the pensioner medical service also became an issue (Sax 1984:61–66).

This system came under widespread criticism in the 1960s for its high costs and gaps in coverage. In particular, it became clear that the commonwealth could not afford to subsidize medical fees that were essentially unrestrained, rising at rates far above those for other goods and services year after year. Reform legislation was passed in 1969–70 to stabilize medical costs through publication of a schedule of fees, to be voluntarily adhered to by physicians (Gray 1991:83–4, 89–91, 96–101). However, this attempt to stabilize medical costs was unsuccessful, and inflated insurance overhead exacerbated the problem. The non-Labor government was unwilling to antagonize its medical allies, and no substantial changes to the system were made until after a change of government in the 1970s.

Non-Labor policy solidified during this period into a position similar to that of organized medicine, supporting predominantly private care arrangements, financed by patient payments and subsidized voluntary private insurance, and supplemented by publicly financed care for the poor. As the opposition party, Labor's general policy came to be the use of government power to deal with vested interests, such as organized medicine, that tend to reduce equality of access or opportunity. In health policy, Labor proposed a universal public health insurance system with controlled medical fees and comprehensive community services, financed by progressive taxation (Sax 1984:75–78, 86–87, 95–96, 100).

Medibank

On December 2, 1972, Labor regained control of the national government. As promised in its campaign, the Whitlam government set out to improve both the organization and the funding of health services by expanding the public role in those fields. New commonwealth commissions were established to plan and implement these programs. For the first time, the commonwealth took a direct role in establishing community health services, including primary care, counseling, disease prevention and detection, rehabilitation, support, outreach, and advocacy. Dental services, mental health, family planning, home assistance, and appliance/equipment supplies were all included, as were local services for areas previously lacking them. All these services were to be funded through targeted and block grants to the states, for both capital and operating project expenses (Sax 1984:102–06).

Labor's initiative, Medibank, represented another major health policy change for Australia. Just as the Menzies government had ended the free hospitalization program put in place by the last Labor government, the Whitlam government ended the non-Labor policy of supplementing private insurance and introduced a universal system of public hospital and medical insurance. Once again, hospital care in the public (now "standard") wards was to be free; in addition, private patients would find their costs lower, as their charges were to become tied to those for equivalent public services. Doctors providing free care to standard ward patients were now to receive salaries, or per-session ("sessional") payments. Medibank medical insurance would allow physicians either to bill the government directly for all their patients at a reduced rate ("bulk billing") or to continue billing their individual patients, who would be reimbursed by the commonwealth (Sax 1984:108).

The success of this insurance program, like that of the previous government, clearly depended on stabilizing medical costs to keep program costs predictable and affordable. Following its successful strategy with the previous government, however, the AMA initiated a series of large fee increases even before the program was passed, forcing the government to request court arbitration three times before Medibank could begin. The medical fees tribunal found twice in favor of the large fee increases requested, and when it found for only a small increase the third time, the AMA refused to accept its decision. Under new trade practices legislation, the AMA could not legally recommend the higher fee increases to doctors; instead, it printed and distributed an "informational list" of fees, showing the same increases the tribunal had denied. This AMA strategy made Medibank both more expensive and less attractive, creating the possibility of large gaps between physician fees and Medibank benefits and reducing the likelihood that Medibank could make most medical care in Australia, for the first time, free at the point of receipt (Sax 1984:110–12).

The government's organizational and funding initiatives were brought to Parliament for passage in November 1973. However, the Senate was controlled by the opposition, and both bills were rejected twice in that body after being passed in the House of Representatives. In accordance with the constitution, Prime Minister Whitlam announced a double dissolution of Parliament, forcing a general election. Organized medicine,

the health insurance funds, and the private hospitals campaigned vigorously against Labor and Medibank, as they had throughout the debate.
Labor was returned to office in May 1974, but it still did not control the
Senate. When a third vote on the two bills ended with the government's
bill being rejected again by the Senate, a joint sitting of the two houses was
convened to deal with the deadlocked legislation, as prescribed by the constitution. This sitting passed both health initiatives in August 1974. The
government's legislation to fund Medibank through a levy on taxable
income, however, was not eligible for consideration at the joint sitting and
remained blocked in the Senate so that the government was forced to use
general revenue funds to finance Medibank (Sax 1984:115–16).

The implementation of Medibank presented still more obstacles.
First, the states had to be persuaded to enter into cost-sharing agreements
with the commonwealth; however, only two of the state governments were
Labor governments, and the non-Labor state governments delayed negotiations and resisted agreement within the terms of the new policy. Furthermore, the private insurance funds refused to act as agents for
Medibank, necessitating the creation of an entire network of new offices,
including agency agreements with retail pharmacies. In addition, although
the AMA could no longer legally advise members to refuse service under
Medibank, it continued to publicly predict delay and failure for the new
system. Many surgeons refused to work on a salaried or sessional basis,
insisting on fee-for-service remuneration and threatening to stop treating
nonemergency public patients. These specialists eventually found themselves in conflict with even non-Labor state governments, however, as the
estimated cost of fee-for-service medical payments was triple that of sessional payments.

Ultimately, the threatened loss of federal funds forced the four reluctant state governments to negotiate agreements with the commonwealth
and institute Medibank in October 1975, three months after its implementation in South Australia and Tasmania (Sax 1984:117–18). In all the
states except New South Wales, physicians agreed to payments by public
hospitals as a part of these negotiations. Many New South Wales hospitals,
however, retained the honorary system (Gray 1990:225).

The Dissolution of Medibank

In November 1975, one month after Medibank came into operation in the
last four states, another stalemate between the House of Representatives

and the Senate prompted the governor general to dissolve the government, ask the opposition leader to form a caretaker government, and call an election. The 1975 election occurred just after the prosperous postwar economy began to falter, issuing in a prolonged period of inflation and recession.

Non-Labor leader Malcolm Fraser campaigned against inflation and high taxes, blaming most of Australia's economic problems on Labor's social programs. In spite of these claims, Fraser promised to maintain the Medibank program if elected. However, once Fraser's Liberal/National Country coalition was elected, economic policy was used to justify immediate changes in Medibank and, over the next seven years, to terminate it altogether. The Fraser government initiated the fourth major change in Australian health care policy and the second non-Labor reversal of Labor-instituted universal public health policy (Sax 1984:126; Gray 1984).

The Fraser government's changes to Medibank were carried out in four sets, with the free hospitalization program lasting through the first three. The first set of changes, only six months after the election, resulted in Medibank Mark II. A levy on income tax, up to a certain ceiling, was introduced to pay for Medibank. Citizens were allowed to opt out of the public insurance system by purchasing private insurance, and doctors were allowed to both bulk bill the government and charge their patients an additional fee. Private hospitalization benefits were added to Medibank, and the government renegotiated the hospital funding agreements with the states to both reduce the commonwealth's share of costs and allow payment of hospital doctors on the fee-for-service basis they preferred. In effect, this first alteration expanded benefits for more affluent citizens, shifted more program costs onto moderate and low-income citizens, and increased the private share of the health care sector, while reducing the commonwealth's expenditures (Gray 1984:5).

A second set of Medibank changes was introduced two years later, abolishing both compulsory health insurance and the levy that had been passed to pay for it. Medibank Mark III substituted a universal subsidy of scheduled medical fees, with higher benefits for pensioners and some disadvantaged groups. In effect, the program remained universal but no longer comprehensive, especially for those moderate and low-income citizens not privately insured. Mark III reduced taxes; however, it also had the unintended effects of increasing both commonwealth expenditures and deficits, while reducing subscriptions to private insurance by the healthy. The resulting problems soon led to a new set of changes (Gray 1984:6).

Medibank Mark V further reduced commonwealth medical subsidies, forcing many citizens to give up their insurance. Insurance companies began to offer cheaper rates for low risk clients, creating even higher costs for other citizens. These changes reduced commonwealth expenditures, but their negative effects on both the private insurance funds and the public prompted intense criticism and a last set of changes (Gray 1984:6–7).

In April 1981, the Fraser government terminated Medibank altogether, returning commonwealth policy to one of subsidized voluntary health insurance and ending Australia's second period of free hospitalization. Commonwealth subsidies were once again limited to the privately insured, the aged, and the poor.

In retrospect, it is not possible to say whether the termination of Medibank was planned by the Fraser government from its election and carried out incrementally or whether the changes resulted from genuine attempts to meet contradictory goals, promises, and pressures. However, the incremental changes in Medibank certainly had the effect of preparing the public for its termination, from the early shift toward private insurance and private care to the reductions in public benefits and the attachment of benefit levels to age and income level. Furthermore, by attaching these changes to fiscal necessity and timing changes to avoid election years, the Fraser government was able to mute criticism and avoid losing office for eight years (Gray 1984). The redistributive effects of Medibank had been limited initially by the failure of the Senate to pass progressive funding; most of its public and decommodifying features were altered within months by the incoming non-Labor government, and the rest were phased out over the next five years.

Medicare

In 1983, however, a Labor government was returned to office. The Hawke government had developed a detailed health policy plan while in opposition and presented it to the public as a major issue in the election. Once in office, the new government moved quickly to reinstate most of the original Medibank program under the new name of Medicare.

Medicare made both standard ward care and outpatient services free to all Australians once again. It reinstated medical benefits at the rate of 85 percent of the schedule fee, with no charge to the patient if the doctor chose to "bulk bill" the Commonwealth Health Insurance Commission, rather than his or her patients. The subsidy of private health insurance was ended and such insurance restricted to coverage of private hospital care and "extra" services, such as dental care. Last, an income tax levy was reinstated to pay for Medicare (Gray 1990:227).

The implementation of Medicare proved far easier than the implementation of Medibank in 1975. For one thing, there were four Labor governments at the state level, so less resistance was encountered from the states. For another, many of the features of Medicare were already familiar from the Medibank program or from their use under the Fraser government. Negotiated ("scheduled") medical fees, for instance, had now become routine, as had the acceptance by hospital physicians of salaries or sessional payments. As a result, the medical profession was less united and less intense in its opposition.

The one major challenge to Medicare, the 1984–85 hospital specialists' strike in New South Wales, ended without significant governmental concessions because physicians were divided, both in their views on Medicare and in their economic stakes in the outcome. The major issue for N.S.W. specialists was the predictable contraction of the private medical market with the contraction of private insurance; however, few other doctors shared their degree of dependence on that market by 1984. State and commonwealth officials were able to make moderate concessions to the AMA, marginalize the more militant specialist organizations, and obtain enough physician contracts to meet the public's hospital needs. In addition, the process was managed in such a way that the outcome was widely regarded as a major defeat for the government, which increased the pressure on the specialists to go back to work (Larkin 1989; McKay 1986; Pensabene 1986).

The literature is divided on whether or not the N.S.W. strike actually represented a victory for organized medicine. However, it is clear that the concessions made by government did not interfere with free hospital care, the trend away from private insurance, or the trend toward physician acceptance of governmental medical insurance payments (Larkin 1989; Chesterman 1986). That is, Medicare retained its decommodifying and public qualities. By these criteria, the N.S.W. strike certainly ended as a victory for Labor policy and state control of the medical field.

Interestingly, neither the private insurance industry nor the private hospital sector was a significant factor in this struggle, although their interests were clearly involved. It appears that neither of these market sectors grew in Australia after 1972 in proportion to its growth in nations with no public health insurance, such as the United States. The most likely explanation of their inaction in this struggle appears to be that both business sectors were weakened by their lack of financial support and inability to compete effectively during periods of Labor policy, producing both less political influence and less financial dependence on tax dollars. The stable medical-insurance-business coalition opposing NHI in the United States has not developed to the same extent, or with the same strength, in Australia.

The Future of Medicare

In 1996, a non-Labor government was elected under Prime Minister John Howard that remains in power today. While the Howard government soon reintroduced private insurance subsidies and reduced regular medical benefits (Sutherland 1997), it has retained many of Medicare's decommodifying and public qualities. Most notably, it introduced a large "concessional" category of Medicare patient, consisting of pensioners, veterans, and means-tested citizens, which receives a higher level of benefits than other citizens (Financing and Analysis Branch 2002). As this category covers a large majority of the population, including both categories of citizen generally considered worthy of public support (veterans, pensioners) and those means-tested citizens frequently demeaned as unworthy, it appears to represent a new approach to NHI in these nations (Light 2002).

That is, previous national policies either have set up separate public programs for veterans, pensioners, and the poor, with coverage reflecting the perceived worthiness of the programs' beneficiaries, or have covered all citizens equally. Furthermore, the simultaneous presence of both public and private health insurance systems in these nations has usually resulted in poor middle- and upper-class support of public systems, resulting in their relative financial starvation. Australia's merging of the special category programs, accompanied by liberalization of the means-test criteria to take in many middle-class families, represents a new compromise, a possible way to destigmatize and maintain majority political support for comprehensive public insurance for all citizens who need it, while allowing more prosperous citizens their choice of either public or private insurance and care.

This shift in non-Labor policy represents a compromise between Labor and non-Labor approaches to health policy and bodes well for the future of NHI in Australia. Interestingly, membership in Australia's trade unions is now rapidly declining, perhaps reflecting a perception that Labor Party strength is less important when non-Labor adopts less extreme positions.

THEORETICAL EXPLANATIONS AND AUSTRALIAN HEALTH POLICY

Political polarization and parliamentary government were identified at the beginning of this chapter as the prime factors in Australian health policy dynamics, which have been characterized to date by extreme swings in policy. However, while Labor governments have consistently moved to change non-Labor health policy immediately upon election, non-Labor governments have clearly felt public pressure to move less quickly in terminating Labor health policy. In addition, while Labor's Medicare program appears to have solidified in a stable and workable form, non-Labor's programs have continued to change in response to problems with inadequate health care protection. More recent swings in Australian health policy have been less extreme than earlier ones, with the policy center moving toward the Labor Party approach. A third prime factor could therefore be said to be Australia's health policy legacy, which has moved national policy increasingly toward more complete health care protection.

Political polarization over Australian health policy, according to power resources theory, would be the result of an effective legacy of working-class organization from Australia's formative period, resisted at every step by conservative economic forces representing the dominant classes. Within this theoretical framework, Australia's legacy of working-class organization constitutes the successful institutionalization of the democratic class struggle through its mainstream Labor Party, national wage boards and Arbitration Courts, strong trade unions, and the working-class consciousness that those institutions both represent and encourage. Political polarization around class issues such as NHI is therefore read as a sign of healthy working-class consciousness and of the use of the political system by subordinate classes to obtain concessions and increase their control over state power resources.

However, class-based political rhetoric in Australia is notably rare and muted, even from Labor Party spokesmen. Political contests play themselves out in terms familiar in the United States: a common interest in national affluence, competing representations of other national and group interests, competing definitions of equality and liberty, controversy over levels of taxation, and electoral appeals to the middle class as the political center. At the same time, state corporate structures have kept the saliency of class-based issues in the public eye, making trade union membership visibly beneficial to workers, with the Australian Labor Party expected to champion worker-friendly legislation and interests. In other words, although political contests are rarely couched in class terms, Australia's institutional legacy builds working-class representation into political discussions so that subordinate class interests are rarely ignored. The fact that many workers frequently support the non-Labor coalition speaks both to the saliency of nonclass issues and interests to workers and to the need of non-Labor to appeal to workers through those issues and interests.

Parliamentary government in Australia has allowed majority votes to translate directly into governmental health policy, in spite of strong minority opposition. The existence of a few constitutional veto points allowed the implementation of NHI to be blocked during early attempts to pass it, but provisions in the constitution for bypassing or altering those veto points eventually ended such vetoes. Specifically, constitutional referendums removed the constitutional barriers, while the provision for joint sessions of Parliament prevented a Senate opposition majority from blocking House majority policy. It is notable that, after the governmental dissolution, election, and joint parliamentary session of 1973–74 over Medibank, such legislative tactics were never again used against Labor health policy.

It is easy to see how political polarization and strong interest-group opposition could have prevented the implementation of national health insurance in Australia, if that nation had the political institutions of the United States instead of its own. First of all, the direct election of a president, separate from legislative party majorities, would have produced executives with somewhat different policy objectives and priorities than the legislative majority, even when both were from the same party. A lack of party discipline in the House and Senate would have left majority-party legislators free to pursue different forms of policy than party leaders. Legislators would then have come under pressure to alter or block leadership programs, as party membership lost its clear connection to either broad or specific national party programs. With no such connection, elections would have become more individualized, with local interest groups gaining more influence in local elections and legislative candidates subject to pressure to alter their support of national party programs in accordance with the wishes of those groups. In essence, each individual legislator would have become a potential veto point for NHI.

This institutionally based blockage arguably could have occurred in spite of the presence of strong social democratic forces. That is, even if trade union and voter support of NHI legislation produced a Labor president, House, and Senate, NHI legislation could still have failed because of preferences or pressures for stronger, weaker, or different health policy legislation. Such divisions would, of course, have been encouraged by NHI policy's opponents, as they are in the United States. In the next election, some individual legislators, or even the president, might have been voted out for their positions on NHI, but no electoral outcome could have guaranteed the passage of NHI or prevented similar divisions and blockages from recurring. In the end, neither the president, legislative leaders, nor individual legislators could have been held accountable for NHI's failure as a whole. The division of political power would have enabled a division of political responsibility, and national elections would have lost their direct connection to particular policy outcomes.

In actuality, however, the prime ministerial system and the tradition of party discipline in Australia have meant that every election of a Labor government from 1940 on has produced a successful governmental effort to pass and implement national health insurance, with increasingly few ways for opponents of such policy to block or alter it. The necessary corollary, of course, is that every election of a non-Labor government from 1940 on has meant a successful governmental effort to institute liberal or market-oriented health policy, with the Labor opposition as helpless to block or alter it as non-Labor was earlier.

In the long run, such policy swings are not necessarily negative. In a politically polarized society, they may allow a policy consensus to emerge from within a wide range of possibilities, unconstrained by institutionally enabled barriers. Logically, a wide range of policy choices is more likely to lead to socially and economically optimal policy than a narrow range of policy choices, constrained by minority obstruction. That is, if a determined opposition can prevent the most workable forms of policy from ever being implemented, a society is forced to make do with less workable forms of policy or with none at all.

In Australia, however, the Labor Party's success at introducing workable forms of NHI appears to have altered the political climate to one in which even non-Labor governments had to accept public responsibility for citizen access to health care and protection from its costs and be prepared to defend the effectiveness of their health policy on those two points. This represents a changed policy trajectory, due to a policy legacy that had proven the ability of government to effectively address these problems.

This policy legacy changed the sense of what government can do in Australia and effectively undermined arguments against welfare state programs. For instance, Medicare has addressed health care needs without stifling Australia's economic growth or increasing inflation, undermining one of the most credible arguments used against NHI from the 1940s to the 1980s. The claim that NHI was bad economic policy relied, in large part, on the relative timing of earlier economic downturns and Labor government programs. As noted, Australia's "free hospital experiment" was ended in the early 1950s by a non-Labor government that came in at the beginning of the prosperous postwar period and remained in power for most of that period. Labor's brief but busy period of government in the early 1970s ended as an economic recession began, a fact that seemed to support non-Labor's economic arguments against Medibank. However, Medicare was implemented in the early 1980s with no apparent negative effects on Australia's economy for a full twelve years. This fact makes it more difficult for the new non-Labor government to terminate Medicare on economic grounds.

In addition, Australia's policy legacy has eroded the influence of entrepreneurial medicine in national policy debates and prevented a powerful for-profit health care sector from developing to oppose NHI politically. Physician solidarity, already somewhat divided by different state policies and medical specialization, has been further fragmented by national policies increasing the number of salaried physicians with interests somewhat different from those of medical entrepreneurs. Use of the strike tactic has called entrepreneurial physicians' professional dedication into question, and their professional claims have been disputed by state and national governments of both parties during conflicts over cost controls. Finally, the referral of conflicts over medical fee schedules to the Arbitration Courts legally reduced such conflicts to a wage and labor issue, placing entrepreneurial medicine's unique claims in conflict with the whole weight of Australia's corporate structure.

Australia's for-profit health care sector has been similarly limited by this policy legacy. The private health care industry in Australia, unlike that in the United States, has not had continuous access to the nation's health care dollars. While often subsidized under non-Labor governments, private health insurance under Labor governments has been denied public tax support, replaced by public insurance, and legally prevented from competing with government programs. These limitations on private insurance have, in turn, reduced the use of private hospitals. Such periods have forced retrenchment in both industries, pushing insurance companies into primary involvement in other types of insurance and some private hospitals into public arrangements. As profit-making opportunities have been limited by such periods, for-profit hospitals remain relatively small, undercapitalized by American standards. Pharmacies remain private, but the prices of essential drugs are subsidized and regulated under governments of both parties, similarly limiting profit margins in that industry. Finally, governmental controls on medical fee inflation have limited the rewards of medical entrepreneurship, resulting in less for-profit experimentation than in the United States.

The result is relatively weak and divided business-sector opposition to NHI. While the for-profit health care sector may strongly desire different policy arrangements, its day-to-day operations require acceptance and self-shaping around existing government policy, which is the primary source of health care dollars. Similarly, its planning process requires the anticipation of future policy arrangements that may further reduce potential profits. Businesses outside the health sector have even less incentive to seek policy changes, and the same day-to-day pressures to accommodate themselves to reality. Active opposition to NHI is quite limited in its effectiveness, as institutional arrangements provide little opportunity for opponents to reverse public policies while a government remains in power. All this limits the potential business benefits of time and money spent on opposition to NHI, and channels most policy-related business-sector activity into negotiations over specific policy provisions.

Business-sector influence on Australian elections appears to vary somewhat with the economy. In practical terms, the large middle class of relatively affluent workers decides elections and therefore receives great consideration from both political parties in all policy matters. In the health care field, this group gets more subsidized private options under non-Labor governments and more protection from economic reversals under Labor. In times of recession, middle-class workers may feel economically vulnerable and vote for more economic protections through a Labor government; it is these votes that business groups have influenced in the past by portraying Labor programs as stifling to economic growth and jobs. In more prosperous times, middle-class workers may desire comforts and options more than guarantees of necessary services; at such times, for-profit health-sector arguments may resonate with a larger segment of the working public, resulting in more votes for non-Labor.

However, other related factors also affect voting behavior. One study has shown, for instance, that public support for NHI programs in Australia has increased after they have been in effect for a while and gone down after periods without them. This suggests that changes in government were only partially influenced by support for health policy issues, since majority support has tended to follow, rather than proceed, policy changes. The same study shows that other welfare state programs were frequently more favored by the public than by government policy (Smith and Wearing 1987).

When other issues have been at the forefront of political contests, health-sector businesses and entrepreneurs have influenced elections by expressing their preferences in terms of other concerns, such as levels of taxation. Their relative weakness, however, limits the amount of influence these groups may wield in Australian politics. Interest-group influence, in general, is also limited by laws that limit the length of electoral campaigns, provide public funding, and require disclosure of large donations to either parties or candidates (Jaensch 1994:48–49, 56). In addition, political ads are banned on television for a short period before each election (Jaensch 1994:59–60). In contrast, trade union representation is built into the Labor Party's structure, assuring regular working-class influence over this major political institution.

In summary, the Australian working class has been fortunate both in the specific form taken by Australian political and electoral institutions and in its early choice of strategies. The parliamentary system has enabled majority rule, while the historic creation of the mainstream Labor Party and a corporate structure for negotiating class conflict have kept working-class issues both in the public eye and in the political process. In the health care area, these legacies and institutions have enabled major policy changes, including some that have built a tradition of state responsibility and have prevented Australian for-profit health sectors from developing the size, strength, and influence of their counterparts in the United States. Despite similar political rhetoric, economic structures, and interest groups to those in the United States, health policy issues in Australia have played out quite differently.

CHAPTER 4

The United States

Attempts to pass national health insurance in the United States have been characterized by political polarization and legislative blockage. Unlike in Australia, where polarization within the parliamentary system resulted in broad national policy swings, polarization within the U.S. political system has resulted in the repeated blockage of NHI legislation and the passage of only a few compromise programs.

Under policies passed in the 1960s, universal government health insurance exists in the United States only for the hospital-based care of the elderly. Federal medical insurance is available to the same group but is not universal, even for the elderly, due to its financing through voluntary individual premiums. The federal government also provides partial funding for state programs for the poor; the Medicaid program, however, assists only a small proportion of those unable to afford health care.

In contrast to Canada and Australia, U.S. proponents of NHI were unable to expand these initial public health insurance programs into universal, comprehensive NHI; the only expansions have been a means-tested program for children and a pharmaceuticals program for the elderly. While state and provincial health insurance programs in Canada and Australia built momentum for a universal federal program, no comparable dynamic occurred in the United States. In the absence of universal public health insurance, the U.S. health care system has become more fragmented, market-oriented, and expensive than that of any other industrialized nation, with multiple gaps in both access to care and financial protection.

HISTORICAL INFLUENCES AND LEGACIES

The United States' colonial period both started and ended rather differently than Canada's or Australia's. For a full century after Columbus' first voyage to the Americas in 1492, European exploration and colonization of the "New World" was dominated by Spain and Portugal, which claimed all the tropical lands considered most valuable at the time. France and England were relatively weak in the 1500s and limited their American activities to exploration and claims in the north, for later exploitation. The European settlement of what is now the United States began with small, scattered English colonies along the eastern coast, the first established in 1607 (Jensen 1968).

Unlike the Spanish colonies, the English settlements were granted royal charters with no financial support; groups and individuals therefore had to bear the costs of colonization themselves. This arrangement inadvertently granted the colonists more political and religious freedom than was common in England at the time as a result of the first colony's business practices; that is, the Virginia Company's rules called for the essentially democratic election of officers and enactment of rules by the stockholders, and prospective settlers were attracted through the promise of company stock. Although the original intent of the company was to control policy from England, colonist discontent forced it to allow the stockholders in Virginia more self-government; these colonists promptly organized themselves as a legislature, modeling their procedures on the British House of Commons. By the time the British government sought to establish political control over the colony, the precedent of representative self-government had been set for newer colonies. Political and religious freedoms therefore became important motives for the founding and populating of the colonies, as well as economic opportunity and the hope of commercial profits (Jensen 1968).

While there turned out to be few sources of quick profit in the North American colonies, compared to the gold and sugar cane of more southern or tropical lands, colonial leaders there recognized the region's great agricultural potential if sufficient farmers and laborers could be attracted. As a result, the colonies were advertised in Europe as regions of opportunity with cheap or free land, and contracts were offered to finance passage to the colonies for those willing to indenture themselves as servants for four to seven years. Over time, the abundant timber, game, and fishing grounds of the North American colonies drew more attention, and the immigration of Europe's landless, unemployed, and entrepreneurial populations grew from a trickle to a flood. The colonies expanded rapidly, and settlers began looking farther and farther to the west for more land (Jensen 1968). Some American colonies received shipments of exiled British prisoners in the 1700s, like those later sent to Australia; however, these penal arrangements occurred late enough to exert little influence on the colonies' development (Sax 1984).

The Seven Years' War, known in the colonies as the French and Indian War, ended with the ceding of French Canada to England in 1763. Britain, in need of funds to replace those expended on the war, sought to raise some through taxes on the colonies it had successfully defended. However, the thirteen colonies were at that time plagued by economic depression, with the colonists feeling hemmed in on the west by British treaties with the Indians and impatient with British interference in general; official responses to colonial concerns frequently took years. At the same time, ideas from the European Enlightenment were circulating in the colonies, providing intellectual and political grounds for challenges to British authority. No longer feeling the need of British protection against French encroachment, the colonies were ripe for rebellion (Agar 1966:3–22; Gay 1968).

The Break with Britain

The First Continental Congress, called in 1774 to coordinate colonial opposition to British "usurpations," issued a declaration of the colonists' rights as Englishmen against a usurping Parliament. By 1776, justification for the rebellion had shifted to the natural rights of man against a tyrannical king in the famous Declaration of Independence, adopted by the Second Continental Congress over a year after fighting had begun in Massachusetts. Four colonies organized themselves as states even before the official Declaration of Independence by adopting state constitutions, a transition that proved relatively smooth. However, arrangements for a coordinating confederation of the states proved so controversial that the Articles of Confederation, approved in 1777 by the Continental Congress, were not ratified by all the states until 1781. Despite this central weakness and considerable opposition within the colonies, the rebels managed to win the Revolutionary War through tenacity, good leadership, and considerable British bungling; Britain recognized the independence of the United States in the Treaty of 1783 (Agar 1966:3–38).

The Articles of Confederation were the work of the more radical democrats in the Continental Congress, who hoped to set up a simple agrarian democracy with weak local governments, and to avoid granting the central authority they were denying Parliament to any American government. Centralization, they believed, would lead to the rule of the rich; sovereignty was therefore reserved to the states, which promptly began erecting trade and other barriers against one another. In fact, so few powers were delegated to the Congress of the Confederation that money could not be raised for the army, foreign debts could not be paid, currency became worthless, and the resulting depression led to farmers' revolts and near anarchy in some parts of the country. The one lasting contribution of the Confederation to the United States was that it convinced all the states to give up their claims to the western lands and agree to a policy allowing those territories to become full partners in the United States as they became sufficiently populated to organize as states. Without that agreement, conflict between the states over the western lands might have prevented the forging of a stronger union in 1787, or the West might have been kept politically and economically subservient to the original eastern states (Agar 1966:25–38).

The Creation of Unique Political Institutions

By 1787, conditions in the Confederation were bad enough that alarmed conservatives were able to convene a convention to revise the Articles of Confederation and then to convince the convention's delegates to produce a completely new document establishing a stronger central government. Regarding the Confederation as a failed experiment, these Founding Fathers saw their actions as a continuation of the Revolution, redirecting it in a more promising direction. They held that "nothing but the first act of the great drama is closed. It remains yet to establish and perfect our new forms of government" (Rush 1787).

With considerable cynicism toward democracy, the delegates set about designing a stable form of government based on the best of the political theories and institutions known to them, especially their own state constitutions, which varied from radical forms with little executive power and no independent judiciary to more conservative parliamentary forms. Ironically, while England was developing the modern parliamentary system of responsible party government later adapted by Australia and

Canada, the American Constitutional Convention was convincing itself that a strict separation of governmental powers was necessary to provide an effective check on the popular branch of the legislature (Agar 1966:39–57).

Eventually, the Constitutional Convention agreed upon a government for which decisive action would be necessarily slow and difficult, deliberately sacrificing efficiency to protect liberty as they understood it. Minorities were believed to require protection from the majority; this would be accomplished in two ways. First, governmental power would be divided among executive, legislative, and judicial branches, with each given some means to check the power of the others. Second, the role of the propertyless in politics would be severely limited by having a president and Senate elected indirectly and by allowing the states to continue restricting the franchise for the representatives of the people. Over time, the second of these arrangements was to be completely reversed, with direct election of the president and Senate and universal adult suffrage. The intentional division of power remained and had an important unintended effect; the government proved so inefficient that it required the informal assistance of political parties to function, an irony because the Constitution's writers thought they had rendered such factionalism unnecessary (Agar 1966).

Labor Development

Organized labor action in the United States preceded such action in both Australia and Canada by several decades, with a first trade union by 1792 and strikes in the 1790s; labor therefore might have been expected to grow into a strong influence on U.S. policies. Indeed, between 1806 and 1842, the early shoemaker and printer labor organizations around Philadelphia and New York were by far the most radical of any in the three nations, defying the combined power of employers and the state in the face of a series of legal prosecutions for conspiracy. However, it was not until 1840 that a single judge in a single U.S. state recognized any right for workers to organize; this Massachusetts judge drew a distinction between the right of workers to organize in the service of their legitimate interests and illegal activities by such legitimate organizations. The right to organize then had to be pursued and fought for in every state. Federal recognition of workers' right to organize was denied by the courts on constitutional grounds throughout the 1800s and well into the twentieth century (Taft 1964).

As in Canada and Australia, U.S. labor organization membership fluctuated with economic conditions, growing in the 1820s and 1830s until the bank panic of 1837, in the 1860s until the 1873 panic, and again in the 1880s. By the 1880s, all the states except Florida had unions, although most were located in the industrial northcentral and northeastern states. The economic crisis of the early to mid-1890s slowed union growth less than previous depressions; it also provoked the development of a farmers' populist political party and marches by Coxie's and other "armies" of the unemployed. As in Canada and Australia, the first U.S. unions were organized among skilled workers along craft lines; unions of unskilled workers along industrial lines did not begin to seriously challenge craft unions in the United States until the 1860s. Early attempts to form U.S. cooperative organizations of multiple craft unions were unsuccessful except for some strike support; it was not until multiple craft unions had formed lasting national organizations that the precursor to the American Federation of Labor (AFL) was founded in 1881 (Taft 1964).

The struggles of U.S. unions in the 1800s centered on wages, the 10 (and then 8) hour day, and working conditions. In its pioneering role, U.S. labor experimented with many forms and tactics. Fraternal benefit associations were organized, as were political organizations addressed to the needs of labor but dominated by middle-class reformers. The importation of cheap or strike-breaking labor through immigration was fought both politically and by organizing immigrant workers. The Knights of Labor, a single broad union for all workers (skilled and unskilled) that advocated producer and consumer cooperatives, was organized in 1869. The Knights of Labor seriously challenged the dominance of the craft unions in several industries and parts of the country until the early 1890s, and its idea of "one big union" was revived in 1905 by the Industrial Workers of the World (IWW) (Hoffman 2001; Taft 1964).

The primary obstacle to U.S. labor success in the early 1800s was a lack of labor rights or legal tools with which to fight violent employer opposition, including the frequent use of police and National Guard or federal troops against strikers. The unions recognized that these obstacles required political action and experimented with both direct and indirect political methods. The first labor party in the world was organized in Philadelphia in 1828 and in New York one year later; the Working Men's parties were unsuccessful at getting their own candidates elected but somewhat successful at electing pro-labor Democrats and getting state

Democratic parties to sponsor prolabor laws. Several other labor parties were founded in the 1800s, the most successful of which was the Socialist Labor Party, founded in 1876. However, these parties were all subject to multiple philosophical splits and tactical disagreements, and those political successes that labor won were achieved more through pressure on the major parties than by labor party electoral successes. By the 1890s, trade union associations were well established nationally and had won support from several presidents and Congresses, but the courts continued to nullify pro-labor executive and legislative acts on constitutional grounds (Taft 1964). The struggle for the legal right to organize and bargain collectively, well over in Canada and Australia by 1900, would not be won in the United States until 1935.

Early Health and Welfare Initiatives

The problems accompanying industrialization and urbanization were acute in the United States by the 1830s; however, the first systematic attempts to address those problems were not made until the 1890s, with the formation of a social welfare reform movement. The movement's members were middle class, driven by the threat they saw to democracy and their own security in increasing extremes of wealth and poverty. Before World War I, this reform movement was divided over the issue of whether specific problems and their solutions were individual or social in nature; much time and energy were therefore spent on forming a coherent set of ideas supporting governmental intervention in matters previously considered individual or private. Nevertheless, some important reforms were achieved during this period. Public health laws were widely revised and extended in the first decade of the new century. Also, the American Association for Labor Legislation (AALL) was organized in 1906 to press for health-related industrial reform. The first campaign of the AALL pushed successfully for Workman's Compensation legislation at the state level, with 41 state programs in place by 1920 (Hirshfield 1970).

As part of the Progressive Party's plank in the 1912 presidential election, reformers put social insurance on the national agenda; by 1913, AALL was ready to launch a state-by-state campaign for compulsory health and disability insurance for industrial workers, based on programs already in place in Europe. Their proposal covered only the lowest paid industrial workers, initially excluding dependents as well as agricultural and domestic workers. By 1917, a model bill had been drawn up adding funeral benefits and dependent health care, and legislation had been introduced in 15 states with initial support from organized medicine, trade unions, a committee of the National Association of Manufacturers (NAM), and other employers (Hirshfield 1970; Walker 1978).

However, this campaign proved far less easy than the one for Workman's Compensation. The state campaigns revealed divisions within AALL over the goals and probable costs of state health insurance, and powerful alliances began to form in opposition to the proposals. Important labor leaders, including Samuel Gompers of the American Federation of Labor, decided that unions needed health insurance as a workplace issue. Simultaneously, a number of employers decided that state insurance was not in their best interests because of the financial contributions they would be expected to make. Commercial insurance companies protested the inclusion of funeral benefits in the model bill, expressing fear that other forms of social insurance might be introduced, competing with their policies or limiting new areas for expansion. The Educational Committee of the Insurance Economic Society therefore targeted the medical profession with inflammatory literature on the possible negative effects of compulsory insurance on physician status and income; this effort paid off in late 1917, when members of several state medical societies refused to ratify their leaders' support of health insurance legislation. At this critical juncture, America's entrance into World War I diverted attention and support from the health insurance campaign. By 1919, state legislatures were unanimously rejecting health insurance. By 1920, the American Medical Association had taken an official stand against state health insurance, and postwar prosperity helped sidetrack social insurance issues by restoring middle-class confidence in America's stability and progress (Hoffman 2001; Hirshfield 1970; Walker 1978).

Federal health care initiatives in the 1920s therefore focused on the shortage of hospitals and doctors and the need for more modern facilities, training, and standards. They did address the health care needs of a few categories of citizens; federal funding for state-based maternal-infant health programs was authorized in 1921, and a medical program for veterans was established in 1924. Experiments in voluntary health insurance began in the 1920s, and it was not until 1932 that governmental health insurance again became a political issue (Hirshfield 1970:28–32; Walker 1978; Anderson 1968:91–103).

DIVISION, DELAY, AND PRIVATE ENTRENCHMENT

Labor Struggles

U.S. labor in the early 1900s was characterized by increasing radicalism, strong reactions to this radicalism, and a resulting division. Immigration continued to provide cheap labor for industrialization while complicating the unionization of the workforce. The labor movement made steady gains in membership, however, especially after the entry of the United States into World War I; organized labor's importance to the war effort was officially recognized by inclusion on several federal wartime committees, and an official Adjustment Commission was set up to arbitrate wartime labor disputes. Much of this union progress was lost at the end of the war, however, when the end of governmental war contracts and the return of millions of unemployed soldiers to the labor market triggered a serious recession. Even after the economy recovered, a wave of labor strikes in the 1920s was largely defeated by determined employers, with police and army support (Taft 1964; Zeiger 1986).

Organized labor was therefore primarily concerned in the 1920s with organizing and workplace struggles, while the AFL maintained a steady effort to obtain the legal right to bargain collectively. Organizers in the mass-production industries struggled to form strong industrial unions in the face of considerable AFL, as well as employer, opposition. The stock market crash of 1929 and subsequent Depression, combined with the Republican administration's failure to address the consequences, resulted in strong worker votes for Democratic legislators in 1930 and for Franklin D. Roosevelt in 1932, the beginning of a long Democratic Party–labor alliance. Congress quickly passed several of FDR's popular relief programs, even though several were controversial within the AFL, which had formed a preference for workplace tactics after repeated political disappointments. One of FDR's relief programs, the 1933 National Industrial Recovery Act, included a section establishing the right for workers to choose representatives and bargain collectively. However, as that act provided no means of enforcement and was declared unconstitutional two years later, the Wagner Act of 1935 was necessary before the right to bargain collectively was finally secured (Zeiger 1986).

The Committee for Industrial Organization was formed within the AFL in 1935. It was made up of a core group of industrial unions that broke away from the AFL in 1938 as the Congress of Industrial Organizations (CIO). Led by John Lewis and the United Mine Workers, the CIO embodied industrial labor's impatience with the conservatism of the craft-oriented AFL, as well as the universal resurgence of labor militance in the 1930s. There were 1,800 work stoppages involving 1.5 million workers in 1934, the most since the early 1920s; union membership rebounded from the losses of the 1920s, tripling between 1933 and 1939 to a new high of 9 million members (Zeiger 1986).

Union growth continued during World War II, reaching 15 million in 1945; however, wartime constraints enmeshed the labor movement in regulatory processes that changed and bureaucratized it. Both the AFL and CIO agreed to forgo strikes for the duration of the war; in return, employers were made responsible for maintaining union membership in all workplaces with union contracts. However, the compulsory arbitration that replaced the strike weapon was considerably slower and less satisfactory to workers, especially in the face of wartime constraints on the right to quit or change jobs. Union leaders found themselves responsible for enforcing both the no-strike pledge and the decisions of the National War Labor Board against their own members. This requirement, combined with "automatic" union membership requirements, reduced many union leaders' responsiveness and closeness to their members, encouraging further bureaucratization and, in some cases, corruption. The result was a larger, but less effective, postwar labor movement (Zeiger 1986).

The New Deal

The Depression had created new pressures for governmental action in several areas, including that of health insurance. President Franklin Roosevelt's Committee on Economic Security (CES) had struggled in 1934–35 with the responsibility of recommending specific welfare reforms, including which social needs to address. A barrage of negative letters from physicians to the CES convinced committee leaders and the Democratic president that a planned, federally subsidized, state-based medical relief program was controversial enough to endanger the whole reform package. As a consequence, health insurance was not included with old age pensions and unemployment insurance in the Social Security Bill of 1935. Similarly, federal funds for state health insurance programs as a part of the National Health Program, embodied in the nonadministration Wagner Health Bill of 1939, were targeted by the AMA; the bill was never referred out of committee for action, and only its public health and children's program funds were later approved through separate legislation (Hirshfield 1970; Walker 1978). The Roosevelt administration was more successful in addressing other Depression-era crises, undercutting popular support in the U.S. for socialist third parties at a critical time for their growth in Canada (Maioni 1998:53)

Depression-era needs for medical assistance in the United States were therefore addressed through a patchwork of emergency and experimental programs, including the rapidly growing hospital-sponsored private insurance plans and more slowly growing medical society–sponsored insurance plans which became the Blue Cross and Blue Shield systems. Legislation to institute compulsory state health insurance was proposed but defeated during the 1930s in Michigan, California, Wisconsin, Massachusetts, and New York. Only New York got as far as a successful vote (a nonbinding referendum), but the start of World War II delayed and eventually killed that proposal. The emergency atmosphere of the war was used to kill a 1941 administration proposal for limited national hospitalization and disability insurance; 1943 and 1944 efforts were equally unsuccessful. However, these attempts represent an important strategic shift by U.S. proponents of public health insurance from state-based initiatives to national proposals; this change in strategy was occasioned by both campaign failures at the state level and Supreme Court decisions indicating that a national program would be constitutionally acceptable (Hirshfield 1970:71–163; Walker 1978; Starr 1982:280).

Approaching the postwar period, then, U.S. health care funding arrangements were both rapidly changing and hotly contested politically, just as in Canada and Australia. Also as in those nations, the primary U.S. political arena for public health insurance moved to the national level in the mid-1940s as constitutionally based objections and obstacles were overcome.

Postwar Unionism

Like Australian and Canadian unions, American trade unions experienced a surge in membership and activism after the war. The implications for national health care policy in the United States, however, were very different.

Both the AFL and the CIO officially formed political action committees in the 1940s, in effect abandoning the third-party option and institutionalizing their alliance with the Democratic Party (Maioni 1998:86). The right for union members to bargain collectively had been won so late in the United States that medical care had already become a hotly contested issue in the battle between employers and unions for worker loyalty; legacies had formed in the mining, lumber, and textile industries of company-run medical services and in the garment industry of union-run clinics and insurance programs. With the 1935 Wagner Act unclear on whether management was required to bargain with unions over health and welfare benefits, unions threw their efforts into winning that battle. This effort was perceived as related to NHI by Walter Reuther and other 1940s labor leaders; they believed that employers bearing the costs of negotiated health insurance would eventually have to turn to the government for relief and work with the unions to pass NHI. By 1954, unions were negotiating one-quarter of all the health insurance purchased in the United States, helping drive the growth of voluntary health insurance there (Starr 1982:311–13; Gottschalk 2000:42–46; Fein 1986:24).

This long struggle, however, diverted union attention and energy away from political action on national policy. While the Canadian CCF and Australian Labor Party were building momentum by 1946 for national health insurance systems through federal subsidies for provincial or state programs, the U.S. labor movement had abandoned the possibility of a working-class party and was struggling for partial control of a growing private health insurance system. The results coincided with other dynamics to alter the organization and funding of health care in the United States, creating the interest groups that would come to exercise such influence there on questions of national health policy.

The Evolution of Private Health Care Financing and Services

The diverse private programs created to insure medical and hospital costs during the Depression evolved in the 1940s in ways that came to dominate the delivery of health care in the United States. These private health plans had actively competed with one another for subscribers and, in proportion to their success, reduced the demand for public programs. At the same time, the specific provisions of the private policies both reflected and increased the involvement of private interest groups. The plans generally fell into one of three categories: indemnity insurance, prepayment plans, or direct service programs.

Indemnity insurance, which reimburses subscribers for covered expenses, was preferred by doctors because it preserved their professional autonomy, keeping the insurance contract strictly between the subscriber and the insurance provider. However, indemnity insurance did not protect subscribers as well as prepayment plans, which guaranteed payment directly to service providers and often covered those costs in full. Since prepayment plans often required providers to negotiate fees, however, most doctors refused to cooperate with such programs unless they were physician controlled. The third category, direct service provision by an insuring organization, was often the most comprehensive for subscribers but also the least controllable by physicians, who were placed more in the position of employees than of independent entrepreneurs. Organized medicine's resistance to prepayment and direct service plans delayed the development of medical insurance for many years (Starr 1982:291–92).

Hospitals' priorities, however, were more compatible with prepayment and direct service plans, and it was their needs that drove the early development of hospitalization insurance. The high cost of constructing, equipping, maintaining, and running hospitals made a dependable income essential for those institutions; for this reason, several individual hospitals experimented quite early with direct service types of programs for large groups, often employee groups such as teachers. In 1932, the American Hospital Association had approved guidelines for acceptable hospital insurance, including a free choice of hospital; city-wide prepayment plans were soon organized to meet these guidelines. Those plans were the beginning of Blue Cross, a national network of state-based, hospital-controlled prepayment plans for nonphysician hospital services. Commercial hospital indemnity insurance was offered once Blue Cross's success appeared assured in 1934; however, commercial companies' contacts with employers helped them catch up rapidly in this field (Starr 1982:295–98; Anderson 1968:119–21; Fein 1986:10–23).

These developments in hospital insurance increased the pressure for physicians to endorse some comparable form of prepayment plan for medical expenses. By the 1930s, about 400 U.S. businesses were providing direct medical services for their employees, and many employee associations had contracts with physicians for prepaid services. In addition, the rural Populist movement had spawned consumer-controlled "medical cooperatives" based on prepayment for services from physicians in group practices. All of these arrangements violated the American Medical Association's 1934 principles of medical service; growing demand, however, resulted in the organization of further departures from the AMA ideal in the form of group practices and prepaid clinics. Organized medicine responded with attempts to outlaw these practices and reprisals against participating physicians, including the loss of hospital admitting privileges, referrals, and consultations. However, patient demand was so great that, in order to suppress alternative programs, some state medical societies finally sponsored their own prepayment plans; these were very successful and became known as Blue Shield plans (Starr 1982:299–310; Anderson 1968:121–22).

The development of private, or voluntary, hospitalization and medical insurance was assisted by state and federal laws passed in the 1930s and 40s to authorize the Blue Cross and Blue Shield systems and then to subsidize its purchase by employers through tax incentives. Heavily influenced by provider and employer interests, these laws shaped the financing arrangements for health care that remain today (Fein 1986:16–26; Anderson 1968:122–23) By the mid-1940s, medicine was increasingly being financed through provider-dominated insurance negotiated with group purchasers of insurance and delivered in group practice settings to meet the prepayment preferences of those purchasers (Starr 1982). While organized medicine jealously resisted the public funding of medical services in the name of physician autonomy, powerful new interests were created through private funding arrangements that would eventually challenge that autonomy.

U.S. HEALTH CARE REFORM INITIATIVES

The Truman Proposal

As of 1945, National Health Insurance had never received clear, public presidential backing in the United States. Democrat Harry Truman reversed this on November 19 of that year with a special health message to Congress. The administration bill proposed comprehensive medical insurance for all classes of citizens, including agricultural and domestic workers, to be paid for by a payroll tax shared equally by employees and employers. Public agencies would pay the premiums of the poor and the unemployed (Starr 1982). Labor had a voice in drafting this bill and provided its strongest support, seconded by the farmer's organization representing the progressive Midwest agrarian movement (Maioni 1998:82–83).

The Democratic-dominated Senate held subcommittee hearings on the bill, planning to provide positive publicity and educate the public on NHI; however, extreme disruptive behavior by some Republican members of the subcommittee successfully diverted media coverage from the bill itself to its opponents' characterization of NHI and its supporters as socialist. After Republicans gained control of Congress in the 1946 elections, the opponents of NHI used new hearings in the same subcommittee to smear NHI as the product of an international Communist conspiracy and to harass supportive witnesses with endless questions on their loyalty and supposed communist connections. In 1947, a House subcommittee held hearings to investigate the participation of federal employees in pro-NHI community workshops; majority committee leaders characterized such federal agency activities as propaganda, an illegal use of federal funds, and part of a Communist conspiracy. Under attack, Truman quietly directed the federal agencies to discontinue their work with pro-NHI community organizations, crippling administration efforts to acquaint the public with the actual provisions of the proposed bill (Allen 1971:81–116).

In similar fashion, every attempt of NHI proponents to publicize their arguments was countered by an extreme and well-funded opposition. When Truman was reelected and the Democrats recaptured Congress in the 1948 election upset, NHI's opponents feared that the administration's bill would finally pass. The AMA responded by assessing AMA members a special fee, hiring the public relations firm that had directed the defeat of the pro-insurance California governor in 1945 and soliciting business and other organizational contributions for a sophisticated anti-NHI campaign. With a virtually unlimited budget and an army of medical volunteers, the Whitaker-Baxter firm saturated the country in a classic campaign targeting pro-NHI legislators and candidates for office, as well as the administration proposal itself, with extreme attacks. Its tactics worked; media support shifted toward the opposition, fewer organizations and individuals testified in favor of the administration bill in the 1949 hearings, and many NHI supporters were defeated in the 1949 elections. By 1950, NHI was abandoned by the administration in favor of an incremental health policy strategy, the unions were focused again on collective bargaining and employer-supplied health insurance, and proponent groups had begun to disband (Starr 1982:286–87; Allen 1971:117–32; Poen 1979; Walker 1978; Gottschalk 2000).

The 1945–49 battle left an important U.S. health policy legacy that profoundly affected future NHI struggles; NHI became ideologically associated with Communism and America's Cold War enemy and therefore politically dangerous to support. This successful political tactic had two important effects. First, public health policy in the United States fell behind welfare state policy in other areas, which were strengthened in the postwar era (Starr 1982:286). Second, the apparent invincibility of the anti-NHI coalition assumed almost mythical status so that health policy proposals were increasingly designed to avoid ideological opposition attacks through limitation to decentralized programs featuring public subsidies of private facilities and services for the assistance of "deserving" groups and persons (Grant 1992). These ideological effects were long-lasting enough that similar arguments and slogans were found in anti-Medicare newspaper editorials and political statements in the 1960s (Behan 1998).

The President's Commission on the Health Needs of the Nation, set up by President Truman in 1951, recommended in its majority report that government encourage universal voluntary health insurance through tax policy, grants-in-aid to the states, and a Social Security–based program for the elderly and disabled. While the dissenting members of the 1932 report had been its conservatives, by 1952 it was the advocates of NHI who were reduced to signing a minority report (Anderson 1968:126–29). As a result, while Australia and Canada experimented with national hospitalization insurance in the 1940s and 1950s, the United States continued to develop a private, profit-based health care system (Walker 1978).

Medicare for the Aged Only

In the postwar period, the United States was characterized by prosperity, nationalism, and optimism. After such wartime scientific successes as radar, the atom bomb, and penicillin, much of the national optimism rested on a strong faith in science; medicine exemplified the basis for that faith with its rapid progress in vaccines and antibiotics. The result was congressional approval of millions of federal dollars for medical research, medical education, mental health programs, and the construction of community hospitals. However, by setting up professional boards whose approval these programs required, Congress established another problematic health policy legacy, one of professional rather than political control over public health care expenditures. Such private control over public funds was unique to the medical policy field. However, these arrangements were not considered controversial in the 1950s climate of exaggerated trust in science and its practitioners (Starr 1982:334–51).

This professional control created a legislative climate in which no health care measure could be passed without AMA or AHA approval. Problematic "gaps" were identified in the private insurance coverage of groups including the poor, disabled, chronically ill, elderly, and rural residents by the late 1950s; it was also clear that much of the private insurance obtained by other citizens provided inadequate coverage of their health care needs (Brown 1956; *New York Times* 1958). However, legislation to comprehensively address these insurance problems was opposed by the AMA, and no such legislation was proposed or introduced by the Eisenhower, Kennedy, or Johnson administrations; several public policies to support voluntary health insurance were proposed instead, and some passed (Anderson 1968). In contrast, when Congress was persuaded of shortages in medical personnel and facilities in the mid-1960s, proposals to address these shortages were passed without difficulty (Starr 1982).

The attention of public health insurance advocates was therefore directed toward solving the health insurance problems of specific deserving groups as part of an incremental NHI strategy. The motivation to begin with the elderly came largely from organized labor, which saw the strategy as a logical adjunct to the employment-related private insurance it was working so hard to build (Fein 1986:54–55; Maioni 1998:108–12). As in Canada and Australia, the first such public insurance policy proposals addressed only hospitalization, which had less political opposition than medical insurance. Unlike in those nations, however, national hospitalization insurance in the U.S. was proposed only for the aged.

The first such proposal, for a program to be run by the Social Security Administration, was introduced by a single congressional representative in 1958; however, the proposal generated such public support, in spite of AMA opposition, that hearings were held throughout the country in 1959. This approach was unacceptable both to the Republican Eisenhower administration and to powerful southern Democrats; however, support grew in both parties as the impact of older voters and the implications of the new proposal became clearer. The chief legislative actor in this drama was Wilbur Mills of Arkansas, chair of the powerful House Ways and Means Committee. In 1960, Mills proposed a far more limited bill establishing the Kerr-Mills program, a state-run program to purchase health care for low-income elderly citizens. Approved overwhelmingly by both the House and the Senate, this program provided partial federal funding for state-based programs (Starr 1982:367–69; Fein 1986:55–60; Anderson 1968:153; Maoini 1998:115).

The Kerr-Mills program was acceptable to the AMA because it would not establish group rights to health services, establish a federal stake in the costs of such services, or interfere with private arrangements for those able to afford them (Starr 1982; Anderson 1968). Three years after its 1960 passage, however, the Kerr-Mills program was in effect in fewer than 28 states and served very few of the elderly there because of limited funds, stringent eligibility tests, and wide variations in types and duration of benefits (*New York Times* 1963b).

President Kennedy therefore introduced the "Medicare" bill in 1961, reviving Representative Forand's 1958 proposal for national hospital insurance for the elderly through Social Security. This bill was reintroduced in every legislative session of his and President Johnson's Democratic administrations until it finally passed in July 1965, after the 1964 Democratic "landslide." Even then, the AMA was able to secure concessions to its interests; Wilbur Mills added a provision to Medicare's public hospitalization insurance provisions, which became Part A, for federally subsidized private medical insurance, which became Part B. This compromise effectively forestalled the future expansion of Medicare to include public medical insurance for the aged by creating an alternative legacy of federally subsidized private medical insurance (Starr 1982:368–69; Anderson 1968:181–93; Fein 1986:60–67; Morris 1985:41–43).

As part of the same compromise, the Kerr-Mills program was expanded into Medicaid, a limited, state-run program to finance health care for the poor. By providing separately for low-income citizens of all ages, this expansion helped forestall the future expansion of Medicare into a universal program (Starr 1982:368–69; Fein 1986:66–67, 129–30; Morris 1985:41–44). This compromise reflected the opposition even within the Democratic Party to a strong, universal welfare state; as a southern conservative, Representative Mills epitomized that opposition.

The Nixon Initiative

The late 1960s and early 1970s saw a rapid increase in the nation's health care costs, encouraged by the insurance arrangements created or won by organized medicine and hospitals through private and public insurance.

No mechanisms had been built into those programs to control prices, and over time, business and government found themselves funding an enormous boom in hospital construction, medical specialization, physician income, and the development of expensive new drugs and medical equipment. As this medical inflation came to threaten other interests with a stake in public and corporate budgets, it began to be taken quite seriously (Starr 1982:380–88; Fein 1986:127; Morris 1985:50).

The political crisis around health care in the 1970s was therefore largely one of costs. At the same time, however, the United States was undergoing cultural and political changes that called attention to inequalities, including those in health and health care. These two concerns came together in a revival of the NHI movement and the adoption of its rhetoric of crisis by business and conservative government leaders (Starr 1982:393).

The revival began in November 1968 with a speech to the American Public Health Association by United Auto Workers' President Walter Reuther, calling for the establishment of a Committee for National Health Insurance to work toward NHI in the United States. The adoption of the rhetoric of crisis began with President Nixon's announcement at a July 1969 press conference that the U.S. medical system faced a massive breakdown if not reformed within the next two to three years. The National Governors' Conference strongly endorsed a proposal for NHI in September 1969. Then a January 1970 cover story in *Business Week* and a special issue of *Fortune* magazine demanded action to reform America's medical system, which was characterized as inferior, wasteful, and inequitable (January 17, 1970:50–64; January 1970:79). For a short time, the policy debate focused on families ruined by health care costs, the maldistribution of doctors and hospitals, and American medicine's failure to keep the U.S. population as healthy as the people of other nations. For the first time, there was bipartisan consensus that new public controls over the health care system would be necessary in order to end the crisis (Starr 1982; Fain, Plant, and Milloy 1977:12; Fein 1986:128–33).

However, the exact reforms needed could not be agreed upon. Senator Edward Kennedy and Representative Martha Griffiths introduced labor's Committee for National Health Insurance proposal in 1970, calling for a comprehensive, federally operated health insurance system with a set national budget and no copayments for health care users (Laham 1992:338–40; Morris 1985:62–63). The Republican administration's counterproposal was based on private insurance through employers and the success of the private Kaiser "health maintenance organization" at reducing medical costs; with a built-in financial incentive for such plans to keep their insured healthy, HMOs appeared to address the concerns of medicine's right- and left-wing critics. However, in adopting this approach, the Nixon proposal critically altered the HMO concept by including several other forms of prepaid care, in particular some "medical care foundations" preserving fee-for-service arrangements; these weakened or destroyed the incentive for good care. Similarly, the Nixon administration introduced rhetorical ambiguity into health policy discussions by characterizing its proposal as NHI, even though the Nixon plan would have consigned low-income families to a separate, less generous insurance program and left an estimated 20 to 40 million Americans completely uninsured (Starr 1982:394–97; Fein 1986:136–37).

The Democratic-controlled House and Senate were unable to agree on either of these proposals; instead, by July 1974, 22 different "NHI" bills were competing for support, including a new, more extensive Republican administration proposal (Laham 1992:340; Fein 1986:146). In April 1974, Senator Kennedy and Representative Mills had drafted a joint nonuniversal "NHI" bill, and by June, representatives of Kennedy, Mills, and Nixon appeared near agreement on a compromise plan. However, these efforts ultimately failed because of opposition from both sides in Congress, including the opposition of organized labor to any plan that represented a reduction in coverage for union families. Labor leaders believed that, in the wake of the Watergate scandal and a national recession, the 1974 and 1976 elections would produce a Congress and president amenable to a less compromised plan (Laham 1992:352–84; Fein 1986:148–49; Morris 1985:76–84; Gottschalk 2000:71). When these predictions were not realized, labor made two important shifts in its policy on NHI. It began to look for an incremental approach to NHI, and it moved away from its strong stand on universalism. By 1978, labor had accepted the idea of employer mandates, or mandatory employer-provided insurance, at least in the short term abandoning decommodification as well as universalism (Gottschalk 2000:75–78).

The only health care legislation finally signed by President Nixon dealt exclusively with the costs of care, through increased controls and mechanisms intended to reduce costs by encouraging competition. This legislation put teeth in a program to control the number of hospitals and nursing home beds, created a mechanism to review the physician-ordered care of hospitalized Medicare patients, and refused payment for those services judged unnecessary. It also provided incentives for training more physicians and mandated the inclusion of HMOs in the benefit plans of larger employers. These policies, for the first time, placed real limits on health care providers in the name of the public good (in this case, the public purse); however, they did nothing to address its inequities (Starr 1982:396–405; Morris 1985:66–76).

Two seemingly unrelated developments during this period had important effects on future health care policy. The first affected organized labor's advocacy of NHI. The Employee Retirement Income Security Act of 1974 (ERISA) was intended to protect pensions by creating federal standards; however, one provision of that act largely exempted employer and union self-insurance plans from state regulation. Broadly interpreted, this provision drastically limited the possibilities for state-level health insurance experimentation and divided workers over discriminatory insurance practices. In combination with the trust funds created by the 1947 Taft-Hartley Act, ERISA created a vested interest for unions in the current system, making them an ally of large corporations in protecting it and creating a split between the interests of unions and nonunionized workers (Gottschalk 2000:39–65).

The second development altered the balance of power between the president and Congress. President Nixon had engaged the Democratic Congress in a struggle over executive versus legislative control of federal spending between 1971 and 1974 by impounding, or refusing to spend, congressionally budgeted funds. These actions were challenged with some success in the courts and were finally ended by the Congressional Budget and Anti-Impoundment Act, which spelled out limited circumstances under which a president could impound funds. The act also created the Congressional Budget Office, increasing the staff available to members of the House and Senate and giving Congress the capacity to conduct independent analyses. Future health care initiatives would find Congress less dependent on the executive branch and therefore even freer to ignore the president's preferences (Morris 1985:51–57).

The Long Hiatus

After Nixon's resignation, President Gerald Ford's first message to Congress included a call for NHI legislation similar to the Nixon proposal. However, economic concerns quickly reduced Ford's support for such a program. Instead, his Republican administration began developing policy proposals that would phase out specialized federal health programs and replace them with block grants to the states. By January 1976, Ford opposed NHI (Starr 1982:406; Ford 1975; Morris 1985:77–85).

Similarly, President Carter ran in 1976 on a platform that included NHI, partly to win labor support; once in office, however, Carter's Democratic administration put hospital cost containment ahead of NHI on its legislative agenda and opposed all but the most limited proposals on economic grounds. The Carter NHI proposal, finally released in June 1979, would have required and subsidized employment-based private coverage for catastrophic illnesses. That coverage would be supplemented by an enlarged public insurance program, replacing Medicare and Medicaid, for eligible individuals not enrolled in private group plans; eligibility would be determined by age, disability, or a means test. The Kennedy-labor coalition supported a more comprehensive plan, also based on an employer mandate and private rather than public insurance; while supported by the AFL-CIO and United Auto Workers, this bill represented a break with previous labor policy that did not go unchallenged. Unable to reach a compromise with Carter, Kennedy submitted a different bill to Congress; due to economic concerns and an impending election, however, neither bill received serious consideration in Congress (Laham 1993:69–81; Starr 1982:411–14; Grant 1992:142; Gottshalk 2000:79–83; Morris 1985:148–71).

With hindsight, it is clear that the nature of the debate over NHI changed during the 1970s, shifting not only toward an emphasis on costs but also toward a more technical debate dominated by budgetary and health industry experts. The concern over costs contributed to this shift, as did the growth in size and complexity of the private insurance and medical industries, along with Congress's increased analytical and bureaucratic capacity. Increasingly, the need for analysis slowed the legislative process, health care bills became more detailed and technical, and moral vision was replaced in legislative discussions by technical language that was nearly incomprehensible to the public (Fein 1986:151–52). In addition, Congress by 1979 had become less dominated by the seniority system and more open to the public, changes that ironically slowed and fragmented the legislative process even further (Grant 1992:159–63). Finally, the technical shift made it more difficult to rally support for specific NHI proposals and answer opposition arguments definitively, while both the technical and institutional shifts increased the difficulties of moving bills through Congress while political conditions were favorable. These trends, as well as labor's discouragement with more comprehensive change, helped make NHI proposals more employment based and limited in scope.

The 1980 election of a conservative Republican president, Ronald Reagan, temporarily ended efforts to pass NHI legislation. Reagan was adamant in his opposition to what he called "socialized medicine"; he had participated in the 1965 AMA campaign to defeat Medicare with such arguments, and had not changed his position since that time (Skidmore 1970:123–38). There was no doubt that the president would veto any pro-NHI legislation that Congress passed; support for Reagan's policies in Congress, however, made any such action extremely unlikely (Morris 1985:172).

The Reagan administration was also opposed to regulation of the health care system, including those efforts begun under the Carter administration to impose systemic reform, cost control, and planning (Laham 1993:82–84). The answer to health cost control for Reagan was to stimulate competition among insurance plans, physicians, and hospitals; in theory, this should force each to practice the economies necessary to offer the best possible services at the lowest possible price. Ironically, putting this policy into practice initiated the intrusive and highly resented regulation of the diagnosis-related group (DRG) payment system. The Reagan administration also reduced spending for targeted health programs, including Medicare and Medicaid, adopting the Ford administration's block grant program. By 1983, the Reagan administration's procompetitive policies were encouraging the corporatization of medicine, another major change in the health care field; however, concerns over equality and quality of care also began to surface, slowing the trend toward decreased federal responsibility in the health care field (Morris 1985:172–88, 212–13; Machado 1985:147–48). Nevertheless, the Reagan administration was successful in keeping health care reform off the national agenda for the duration of its term of office (Laham 1993:84).

In 1988, Reagan's vice president, George Bush, was elected to the presidency. As a candidate, Bush promised not to raise taxes, a promise that precluded NHI; as president, Bush continued the Reagan administration's health care policies. Because of medical inflation and increasing gaps in private health insurance coverage, however, NHI reemerged in 1991–92 as a national political issue. One important factor in this dynamic was economic recession; a newer factor was the global economy, which was increasingly being used to justify corporate layoffs. As more workers suffered periods of unemployment and found themselves reduced to working for small employers offering few or no insurance benefits, middle-class families increasingly found themselves without health care coverage (Laham 1993:90–95). The number of uninsured Americans increased from 33.6 to 35.4 million between 1988 and 1991 (Aaron 1991:74). By 1990, 70 percent of the uninsured were in year-round, full-time working families, 44 percent had incomes of over $20,000 a year, and 27 percent earned over $30,000 a year (Kosterlitz 1992:385).

Workers who retained corporate positions were affected as well; as the cost of health insurance benefits to employers continued to rise, many large companies increased the share of the insurance premium borne by employees and adopted plans that increased the out-of-pocket costs of care through deductibles, copayments, and exclusions. For similar reasons, Medicare premiums and deductibles had been steadily rising for decades; between 1965 and 1992, the share of the elderly's income spent on health care had risen from 15 to 19 percent, a larger share than before Medicare began. As the threat to middle-class individuals and families grew, so did public support for fundamental health care reform (Laham 1993:95–98).

In November 1991, a political unknown defeated Pennsylvania's former governor for a Senate seat on the issue of health care reform, over-coming a 44 percent gap in the polls (Kramer 1991; Hertzberg 1991). Facing a reelection campaign in 1992, President Bush belatedly promised to introduce a health reform plan. His plan, announced in February 1992, proposed a system of tax deductions or tax credits to reduce the cost of pri-vate health insurance for families not covered by Medicare or Medicaid; he proposed cuts in Medicare and Medicaid to finance this program. In addi-tion, Bush proposed the creation of large networks of small businesses to purchase group health insurance for their employees, voluntary measures to reduce insurance paperwork and encourage enrollment in HMOs, and legislation to discourage malpractice suits. Congressional Democrats attacked this plan for its failure to provide effective cost controls or uni-versal coverage; when President Bush refused to negotiate over the pro-posal, NHI was effectively dead until after the next election (Laham 1993:126–40).

The Clinton Proposal

President Bill Clinton was the first president since Carter to be elected on a platform including NHI and the first since Truman to send a proposal for comprehensive, universal NHI to Congress. President Clinton made

NHI a priority of his first administration, putting first lady Hillary Clinton in charge of his task force on health reform and introducing the resulting Health Security Act to a joint session of Congress on September 22, 1993. The timing appeared favorable for action, with a strongly Democratic Congress and continuing changes in the job market generating middle-class anxiety about costs and access to care. In addition, employers were quite concerned about health care costs, and the Clinton proposal adopted their preferred approach, dealing strongly with both costs and access. However, the bill's introduction was delayed by other priorities, as was the administration's effort to explain it to the public, while its opponents had begun organizing to fight it long before it was completed. Although public support was initially strong, and legislators of both parties promised to work together to solve the problems it addressed, in the end, the Health Security Act suffered the same fate as its predecessors (Laham 1996; Skocpol 1996; Mintz 1998; Blankenau 2001).

Although its name was borrowed from the 1970 and 1974 bills proposing a public insurance system, the Health Security Act was actually a complex variation of the compromise plan based on employer mandates that had been rejected by labor in 1974. The Clinton proposal required states to establish regional alliances to contract with private insurance carriers for plans meeting certain standards; these would create large insurance pools and maximize competition to keep costs down. Insurers would be required to accept all alliance members at community-based rates without excluding preexisting conditions; the resulting reduction in administration would help reduce costs, as would a cap on insurance premiums tied to the Consumer Price Index. Employer concerns were accommodated with both limits on their costs and a provision allowing large employers to opt out of the regional alliances. The bill provided funds to subsidize the premiums of low-income families and to cover Medicaid recipients through the same alliances (Laham 1996:29–36; Hage and Hollingsworth 1995; Skocpol 1996; Gottschalk 2000).

The bill was a compromise between the employment-based private insurance system favored by conservatives and Clinton's goal of universal coverage. Its cost-control measures were necessitated both by the president's promise not to raise taxes and by laws passed in response to the Reagan deficit. It represented a form of NHI that would have been redistributive, but not decommodifying, and would have increased public control of the health care field without an additional infusion of public funds. As such, the plan both antagonized supporters of a stronger form of NHI and faced determined opposition from antigovernment conservatives, noninsuring employers, smaller insurance firms, and other health care stakeholders that feared the bill's effects on future profits. Furthermore, the complexity necessary to meet so many competing demands made the bill confusing, creating uncertainty among its potential supporters and opportunity for its opponents (Gottschalk 2000:65, 137–58; Mintz 1998; Skocpol 1996).

The legislative sticking point for all NHI proposals to date had been congressional committees, which provided delay while opposition arguments were mustered and competing measures introduced; given enough delay, public support could be diluted, and other priorities would intervene. As useful veto points, congressional committees command much attention from interest groups that fear legislative action, including representatives of the health industry (Laham 1996:41–63). As the momentum built from 1991–93 for health reform legislation, health industry donations to the campaign funds of members of the committees and subcommittees with responsibility for health care bills rose substantially (Rubin 1993).

With access to such influential legislators, its opponents were able to significantly delay action on the Clinton proposal; in the meantime, a massive public relations effort by the health insurance industry and the Republican opposition, which seriously misrepresented the Health Security Act and its probable effects, was successful in reducing its public support. Business, which had initially offered some support for health care reform, united during this interval against the Clinton proposal. Labor was divided and largely ineffective in its support. By August 1994, health care reform bills had been voted out of three of the five necessary committees, too late for either house to reach agreement on a bill before the end of the legislative session. No floor vote on any health care measure was taken (Laham 1996; Hage and Hollingsworth 1995; Bergthold 1995; Gottschalk 2000; Skocpol 1996; Mintz 1998). Once again, all the public concern and support and all the presidential and congressional efforts made to pass comprehensive health policy legislation had come to nothing.

In 1997, however, a much less ambitious new means-tested public insurance program was passed with the president's support. The State Children's Health Insurance Program (SCHIP) offered grants to the states to provide health insurance for uninsured children whose families are not poor enough to qualify for Medicaid. States could use the funds to expand Medicaid or to set up a separate program for eligible children, based on either public or private insurance. Within three years, all fifty states had passed programs to utilize the available federal SCHIP funds (American Academy of Pediatrics 2000). In general, SCHIP insurance is less comprehensive than Medicaid insurance, less expensive for the states, and serves a somewhat older and healthier category of children (Byck 2000). While many SCHIP programs are still developing, research has already begun to document the usual problems with means-tested programs in the United States, that is, gaps in coverage and declining financial support, particularly when budgets are tight (*Mental Health Weekly* 2002; *AHA News* 2001).

Most recently, under a Republican president, a Republican-dominated Congress passed the 2003 Medicare Prescription Drug Act. This bill alters Medicare by adding provisions for voluntary prescription drug insurance and other market-based options, including larger subsidies for private insurance alternatives to traditional Medicare. Many of the bill's provisions will not go into effect until 2006, and some of its implications are not yet clear (Hurley and Morgan 2004; Pear 2003; Kemper 2004). However, as with the SCHIP bill, the Medicare reform bill combines addressing a U.S. health financing gap with incentives to further shrink public health insurance; its sponsorship by anti-NHI political forces attests to its expected effects. The bill may face revision before it fully takes effect, as legislators of both parties have become concerned about its potential for increasing both future health care inflation and federal budget deficits. Its provision prohibiting Medicare from negotiating with drug companies for volume discounts prompts the first concern, and the discovery that the administration's original estimates of the program's costs were far too low prompts the second (Pear 2004; Sherman 2004; Weisman 2004).

Because of their provisions for shrinking public health insurance, neither the 2001 SCHIP nor 2003 Medicare bills appear likely to help move the United States closer to NHI. If they should eventually do so, their contributions will most likely have been the broadening of the categories of citizen and health services for which the public expects government to assure access.

THEORETICAL EXPLANATIONS AND U.S. HEALTH POLICY

The history of health policy in the United States calls attention to several dynamics. First, there is the clear importance of political institutional obstacles to comprehensive policy change, even when the president and a majority of the members of both houses of Congress publicly support such legislation. Unlike in Canada and Australia, strong executive and legislative support does not guarantee legislative action. Considering the evidence that the writers of the Constitution introduced such veto points intentionally, this fact is not surprising.

These unique political institutional obstacles appear to have resulted from the timing and manner of the U.S. break from Britain, combined with the failure of the first, arguably more democratic, U.S. central government arrangement. That is, since Britain's development of responsible party government occurred after 1776, but before Canada or Australia became independent, the timing of the U.S. separation from Britain appears to be one critical factor in its unique institutions. In addition, the American colonies' violent separation from Britain created conditions there that did not favor the adoption of British institutional innovations, as did conditions in Canada and Australia. Finally, the failures of the initial, radically decentralized U.S. Confederation in conducting the nation's business appear to have motivated the Constitution's writers to move in the conservative direction of a separation of federal powers, rather than a direction that placed more trust in democratic decision-making; those failures may also have convinced the thirteen state legislatures to ratify the rather antipopulist results.

Second, U.S. health policy dynamics call attention to the lack of consistent support from organized labor for NHI and to the failure of labor parties to thrive in American politics. The early U.S. labor movement's expressed disappointment in the political system and the results of its political efforts appear to support the contention that U.S. labor turned from political to workplace efforts to obtain health insurance because of political institutional dynamics that favored the blockage, rather than the passage, of NHI. Similarly, efforts to organize a mainstream labor party appear to have been largely scuttled by the relatively early organization of the Democratic and Republican parties, their broad nature, and their central role in the functioning of the federal government. However, the Canadian CCF/NDP has survived in spite of the same difficulty there, through the development of provincial parties and the election of third-party provincial governments; tensions between provincial and federal governments within a system of responsible party government, absent in the United States, may have facilitated that survival in Canada.

Third, U.S. health policy dynamics call attention to the increased influence of interest groups there, particularly in their ability to get legislation blocked or weakened. While organized medicine and business vehemently opposed NHI in all three nations, these interests were only able to block legislation in the United States. This is compatible with one of the theoretical presumptions of this book, that interest groups gain influence on this issue only when class politics are blocked or made institutionally untenable.

Class dynamics in the United States were similar to those in Canada and Australia in the steady growth of the trade union movement, except during most periods of economic depression, until the 1970s. They are clearly different in the lack of an effective national labor party and in the repeated blockage of working-class friendly legislation. The pioneering role of U.S. labor in the worldwide labor movement is not fully appreciated in the United States, and that very pioneering may have led to some errors from which other labor movements were able to learn. However, between the courts and Congress, labor rights were exceptionally slow to be recognized in the United States, a fact that calls our attention again to U.S. political institutions.

In addition, while working-class issues such as NHI have been championed by the CCF/NDP in Canada and the Labor Party in Australia, they have primarily relied in the United States on the Democratic Party, a political party long split by its representation of both trade unions and southern conservative elites. This split was facilitated, in turn, by racial divisions within the labor movement and the country in general. The split within the Democratic Party led repeatedly to the introduction of NHI legislation by Democratic presidents or legislators, followed by its blockage by southern Democratic legislators in key committee positions.

Class dynamics around NHI have also differed in the United States through congressional institutional change. Without responsible party government, dissatisfactions with and within Congress have focused on a tradeoff between efficiency and democracy, rather than challenging the fragmented nature of legislative power. That is, the direction of change has either been to promote efficiency by extending the means to build individual power bases within the House or Senate through seniority, committee assignments and chairmanships, or to attack those arrangements because of the opportunities they create for corruption and abuse. Either way, the obstacles to class-based legislation are not reduced;

efficiency through powerful individuals creates powerful veto points, but a lack of powerful individuals in such a fragmented system makes the negotiations necessary to pass comprehensive legislation nearly impossible.

Furthermore, campaign contributions naturally flow to such powerful legislators from interest groups desiring their assistance, a dynamic that systematically favors groups controlling significant wealth over those that do not. Democrats, traditionally disadvantaged in raising campaign funds in comparison to Republicans, have as incumbents enjoyed their ability to command significant interest-group donations and therefore have not acted vigorously to reverse these arrangements when in power. The lack of an established class-based party has then meant that there has been no strong and consistent voice condemning this dynamic, which has produced repeated delay, obstruction, and failure to act on pro–working-class legislation and to obfuscation of the issues through multiple competing bills and the avoidance of floor votes.

This dynamic has, in turn, produced discouragement and a retreat from class politics among American workers. The failure of pro–working-class legislation has repeatedly convinced labor activists and leaders to look elsewhere for solutions to working-class problems. The participation of the organized working class in elections has waned, reducing the rewards for politicians who champion working-class interests and the risks for those who ignore or oppose them. As a consequence, the influence of active interest groups over class-based legislation has grown, especially those advocating the interests of elites. In the medical field, the lack of NHI has allowed the development of a uniquely large and powerful U.S. private health care industry. As an organized and well-funded interest group, this industry is able to exert considerable influence over any legislation that might affect it, including NHI.

The dynamics that occur around class-based legislation in the United States are then dominated by the interests of key political players and interest groups. Key political players are determined chiefly by institutional position, with the occasional exception of a player whose influence depends on interest, expertise, and public recognition (i.e., Senator Edward Kennedy).

Key interest groups, then, are determined by their ability to influence key political players through campaign contributions and lobbying, the organization of "grassroots" letter campaigns, public relations campaigns directed toward the public, or all three. Such activities are chiefly limited by the availability of funds, although an extraordinarily committed working-class interest group may achieve some influence by flooding Congress with letters or voting as a block, as members of the religious right occasionally have done. As this dynamic has matured, public relations companies have developed that specialize in influencing Congress and the public on political issues. As the effectiveness of such companies has grown, the relative financial disadvantage of working-class organizations has come to be a larger factor in political action.

The acceptance of interest-group activity, rather than class-based activity, as the norm in American politics has resulted in the perception of the labor movement as just another interest group, with no broader or more representative perspective than any other group. Corporate influence has then been justified as necessary to balance the influence of organized labor, in spite of the enormous resource disparity between the two groups. Finally, Supreme Court decisions have upheld these arguments, increasing the difficulties of renewed class-based political action in the United States as compared with Australia or Canada. This analysis finds the historical evidence consistent with the premise that interest groups have acquired disproportionate political influence over national health policy in the United States because of the institutionally based blockage of organized working-class influence.

CHAPTER 5

A Second, Systematic Approach

THE THEORETICAL IMPLICATIONS OF THE THREE NATIONAL STUDIES

The findings in the traditional comparative historical studies appear to support the premise that NHI is a class issue, which requires power resource variables to explain. They also appear to support the premise that political institutions differentially affect national social democratic dynamics in these nations, and are compatible with the idea that interest groups assume more power over such issues when working-class organizations are divided and their goals blocked by hostile political institutions. These results can be elaborated theoretically as follows.

The political struggle for national health insurance, like those for all welfare state policies, is part of the wider democratic class struggle (Esping-Andersen 1990). The democratic class struggle concept accepts Karl Marx's premise that the working class is subordinated in capitalist societies and posits that this class's disadvantage in power resources, in relation to those of the capitalist class, can be decreased through collective action focused on political control of the state (Korpi 1983). Within Sorensen's formulation, this premise treats class in its exploitive sense, positing that what is good for the dominant class in a capitalist society is frequently at the expense of the working class and that this fundamental difference in interests underlies class conflict (2000).

Applied to health care, this premise notes that when both health care and labor are treated as commodities, with their value determined solely through market forces, health care becomes unaffordable for many members of the working class. Lack of access to health care, through adequate wages or as a benefit of employment, threatens both the length and the quality of working-class families' lives. Access to health care in capitalist societies is, therefore, a problem for members of the working class. In precisely the same way, when health insurance is treated as a market commodity, financial protection from health care costs becomes unaffordable for many workers. This arrangement favors the dominant classes[1] by forcing workers to stay in the labor market and compete for the better rewarded jobs. Legislation addressing this issue in these nations has two necessary characteristics; it must be decommodifying, and it must be public (Esping-Andersen 1990), for the following reasons.[2]

Legislation making either health services or health insurance available to all citizens through the state is decommodifying because it effectively removes access to such care and insurance from the marketplace. Such policies establish a social right (Marshall 1964) to health security for all citizens regardless of ability to pay and reduce the commodification of labor by separating access to health care and financial protection from employment and the labor market. The withdrawal of one's labor then involves less risk of an uninsured health emergency and becomes a more viable worker strategy in the struggle for good wages and working conditions. National health insurance is, therefore, decommodifying in nature, and its passage reduces a dominant class advantage over workers in capitalist societies.

NHI also incorporates the financing of health care into the public or democratic realm, creating a policy legacy that ultimately reduces the dominance of the private or market realm over health care arrangements. That is, the costs of health services and insurance become public issues once responsibility for their financing moves to the state, and arrangements which increase those costs may be legitimately questioned. Decision making that favors private advantage or profits is seen as less legitimate in the public realm than in the marketplace, and standards such as public benefit may be applied. State legislation instituting NHI therefore introduces a basic shift in health care arrangements from private to public decision making.

Such a shift is in the interest of the working classes, which constitute a numerical majority in all industrialized societies; to the extent that democracy represents majority rule, workers should be able to influence decisions in the democratic state, while they exercise no comparable influence in the market. Such legislation therefore constitutes, at the most basic level, the use of the democratic state to limit the power of capitalism over workers' lives, altering the power differential between the dominant and subordinate classes.

However, the extent to which a nation's NHI is decommodifying and public is variable, and that variance can be measured. For instance, some nations establish two-tier systems of health financing that are minimal for their poorer citizens but generous to those who can pay contributions or user fees. In such a system, optimal care remains commodified. However, if back-up systems of insurance for the unemployed are provided, employment may determine the comprehensiveness, convenience, or comfort of care but not access to its basic forms. This connection keeps some pressure on workers to compete for jobs but less than if basic access were at stake.

In addition, the public/private mix of NHI programs varies. Some forms of NHI are completely public, leaving no role for private or market insurance organizations. In other forms, the state organizes the provision of health insurance through private insurance providers or subsidizes the purchase of private insurance. Clearly, a program which institutionalizes a role for private insurance companies establishes a different policy legacy than programs that shut such agents out; one legitimates the role of private insurers, while the other delegitimates them. In different words, one cuts the connection between private insurance and health care altogether, while the other compromises between the market interests of insurers and the public's interest in having every possible health care dollar spent on actual care. Totally public systems therefore legitimate more democratic decision making about health care arrangements than programs with market components and represent a more effective use of democracy to limit the power of capitalism in workers' lives.

For all these reasons, both the passage and the form of national health insurance are properly regarded as class issues. It follows that the question of why a single industrialized democratic nation has not instituted NHI necessarily involves the question of why the workers in that state have been unsuccessful at translating their numerical strength into worker-friendly legislation. This question suggests the need to consider nonclass factors which influence class-based legislation by affecting the ability of the working classes in different nations to organize and act effectively.

Political institutions have this capability. Political institutions shape the ability of political actors to organize and advocate specific types of policies, making the effectiveness of citizen mobilization contingent on formal and informal institutional processes of politics and governments (Immergut 1992b). In this way, the rules of the game defined by political institutions in some nations may increase the impact of subordinate-class actors, linking the interests of the working class to policy outcomes. In other nations, political institutions may reduce the ability of working-class organizations to realize their goals.

Specifically, political institutions can affect the capacities of working-class actors to influence health policy in at least two ways. First, constitutional arrangements for responsible party government, cabinet coalitions, and multiparty systems heighten the salience of class divisions and encourage the emergence of class-based parties in liberal nations. Broad, class-based interest groups with strong ties to partisan political parties emerge where rules for elections and governing allow groups and parties to advocate class-based political positions and realize their goals once in power. In contrast, winner-take-all elections and fragmented power encourage the formation of two ideologically broad political parties containing multiple, narrow interest groups. These allow political minorities to block legislation, reducing the ability of working-class advocates to realize their goals and shaping different political outcomes.

As a case in point, Ellen Immergut describes how the alteration of political institutions in Sweden, negotiated during the transition from monarchical to parliamentary rule and the extension of the franchise, had unexpected consequences favorable to social democracy. Divided rule, at first between the monarch and Parliament, and then between an indirectly elected First Chamber and a directly elected Second Chamber, resulted in the evolution of a mediating system that allowed policy making to proceed smoothly. When proportional representation helped the Social Democratic Party win an unexpected 1932 victory, and that party allied with the Farmer's Party for a stable majority in both chambers, all the "veto points" with which the parliamentary minority had been able to block the programs of the majority were suddenly removed. Executive decisions were translated smoothly into law, and the Social Democrats began 44 years of uninterrupted rule. NHI was instituted in 1946 (1992a:179–90).

In contrast, Steinmo and Watts describe how U.S. Medicare was shaped by constitutionally fragmented authority, congressional committee prerogatives, an ideologically divided Democratic Party, and repeated failures to move health reform legislation to passage in spite of strong public support during the Roosevelt, Truman, and Kennedy administrations. Intended by its authors as the first step in an incremental strategy towards

NHI, Medicare was altered by the conservative chair of the House Ways and Means Committee, Wilber Mills, in ways that undermined its future expansion. The price of universal public hospital insurance for the elderly was an arrangement that pitted those in need of public insurance against one another for program dollars, inflated health care costs, and utterly failed to confront problematic aspects of the American medical industry (1995:346–50).

Political institutions can also affect the ability of class actors to affect health care policy in a second way, through the institutionalization of class-based political divisions. That is, political traditions or legacies of organization around class divisions create conditions advantageous to the passage of NHI; for instance, labor parties keep the need for worker-friendly legislation on the political agenda and problematize attempts to block it. Such traditions can lead to the institutionalization of state-sponsored, class-based negotiations over proposed policies, that is, "corporatist" arrangements. Formal corporatist arrangements for national-level bargaining between capital and labor encourage class solidarity by increasing the political salience of class interests relative to other interests. Such arrangements both legitimate and provide a forum for articulating class-based demands such as NHI.

In contrast, the lack of such arrangements increases the influence of narrower interests in government programs by limiting organized working-class input and aggravating divisions within that class. Political interests then become organized and actors mobilized around narrower-than-class interests. The relationships between subordinate-class groups necessary to social democratic struggle are not forged, and intraclass divisions are engendered by pluralistic struggles, as when communities organize around competition with one another for factories and jobs. As institutional arrangements that affect the ability of the working class to affect policy, political legacies and state corporatist arrangements overlap with constitutional electoral and governing arrangements.

For instance, Sweden, under the unimpeded rule of the Social Democrats, instituted a formal corporatist arrangement of the type described above. Under these political conditions, the welfare state negotiated was extremely generous, promoting an equal, high living standard for all; Norway and Denmark instituted similar arrangements. Under different political conditions, nations have organized class interests very differently. In Austria, France, Germany, and Italy, for instance, corporatist arrangements were shaped by the Catholic Church and by Christian democratic, rather than social democratic, political traditions. These welfare states tend to uphold status differences by attaching different levels of state benefits to class-specific arrangements and preserve traditional families by treating many state services as subsidiary to the family's duty to care for its own. As a result, social rights are uncontested in these nations, but their decommodifying impact is very small (Esping-Andersen 1990).

A third group of nations, of which the United States is the most extreme, tends to deny broad class interests and treat class organizations as just another "special interest." With neither a class-based political legacy nor the church-based corporatist arrangements described above, class advocates in such "liberal" nations struggle for legitimacy, and broad class interests compete with narrower interests for the attention of the media, political parties, and elected leaders (Esping-Andersen 1990). Under such arrangements, members of the dominant class can effectively represent their class interests through business, civic, and partisan interest groups, but members of the working class, with less access to resources and policymakers, struggle to mount a response (Domhoff 2002). The result can be a labor movement that largely gives up on class-based public initiatives and concentrates instead on building a partial, private welfare state for organized workers through partnerships with employers (Gottschalk 2000).

From the perspective of this work, then, policy outcomes emerge not only from the demands of various groups but also from procedural mechanisms that determine how demands are voiced and what types of groups make them (Immergut 1990). Such procedural mechanisms may not be as important where working-class forces are well organized and strong; in the face of weaker class forces, however, procedural mechanisms may be decisive in determining the viability and form of national health policy. Therefore, political institutional factors are necessary but not sufficient to explain the fate of NHI proposals; class factors are also necessary.

This elaboration incorporates insights from three of the theories discussed in the introduction. From political institutional theory is taken the importance of institutional structures and legacies, their impact on actors' goals and strategies, and their role in shaping the policy outcomes that create new structures and legacies. From power resources theory is taken the central concept of the democratic class struggle, NHI's objective significance in that struggle, and its relation to majority versus minority rule. Finally, from pluralist theory are taken the dynamics that replace majority rule in nations with weak class organization and divided political power, creating multiple points where legislation may be altered or blocked. This elaboration integrates the three approaches by identifying the role of institutional context over time in shaping and constraining class and interest-group goals and successes and by tying the effects of the resulting political legacies to national health policy.

A SYSTEMATIC COMPARATIVE HISTORICAL METHOD

The studies of the three nations' health policies, as presented in the past three chapters, appear to support the theoretical conclusions elaborated above; however, as noted before, the results of traditional comparative historical research may reflect investigator bias in the selection and/or interpretation of historical materials. For that reason, a second, more systematic comparative historical method was used in this study to check and expand on the results of the traditional analyses. Carefully conducted and reported, this approach should provide readers with the information they need to evaluate the traditional study results.

This systematic method, qualitative comparative analysis (QCA), also provides a way to test for the harder to recognize causal patterns. This is useful, because complex phenomena such as national health policies appear unlikely to result from a single necessary and sufficient cause. It is possible that they may be determined independently in different times or places by any of several sufficient factors (multiple independent causation); it is also possible that they only occur when several necessary factors overlap at the same time and place (conjunctural causation). Either of these patterns would explain a good deal of the theoretical confusion over this issue, and only a method that tests for all of these possibilities can offer a definitive answer.

QCA Dilemmas and Solutions

In traditional comparative historical analysis, nations are generally treated as the "cases" of a phenomenon to be compared. However, it would be problematic to use this approach in a study investigating three nations, with one constituting the only negative case, as this would make the logical elimination of spurious causes quite difficult. That is, many possible causal factors are likely to be identified within the two nations showing positive outcomes, but the limits of the single negative case may make it impossible to eliminate those factors which are not causal. This is notably the case with U.S. exceptionalism, where several of the factors that have been identified as important to the passage of NHI in other countries—types of state institutions, political parties, labor movements, national cultures, and so on—are either absent, considerably weaker, or appear qualitatively different in the United States (Steinmo and Watts 1995; Navarro 1989; Lipset 1989).

One solution is to expand our definition of cases to include time periods as well as countries, creating negative and positive cases within a single country at different times, as well as negative and positive cases within different countries at similar times (Orloff 1993; Skocpol 1984). This is probably the best single solution if our phenomenon of interest is a single phenomenon, easily identified and agreed upon as present or absent in a particular time and place.

However, national health insurance programs have been implemented in different nations in multiple forms, and there is little agreement on what constitutes the essential elements of NHI. For instance, some forms include all citizens, others include all resident citizens and noncitizens, and still others include only those resident citizens qualified by some criteria. Even if all social scientists were to agree that NHI is defined by the quality of universality, no agreement exists at present as to what constitutes universality. Similarly, even if we agree that NHI must, at a minimum, guarantee all citizens access to health care and protection from health care costs, there is no agreement as to what constitutes reasonable access or financial protection. Therefore, our phenomenon of interest, NHI, is a disputed rather than easily identified and agreed upon phenomenon, and the designation of positive and negative cases can be expected to be controversial.

Another solution to a lack of negative cases appears to avoid this difficulty; it is to use Tilly's distinction of different types as providing negative cases for each other (1984). That is, the qualities of interest in national health insurance programs can be delineated and used to distinguish different types of national health policy from among a range of nations, including the United States. These types can then be used as negative cases for one another and correlated with possible causal factors. For instance, instances of political initiatives resulting in national health policy addressing basic care for citizens poor enough to pass a means test ("residual" type outcomes) may be used as negative cases for those instances that resulted in comprehensive health insurance for most citizens ("decommodifying" type outcomes), and vice versa. The causal factors correlated with each type of case can then be compared with one another.

This solution offers the advantage of allowing the researcher to specify what is found and then suggest and defend logical typifications of those findings, rather than to use and assert agreement on larger nominal categorizations, such as NHI, that are in dispute. This offers, in effect, a middle-range method for building middle-range theory.

Notably, both solutions can also be used in combination. That is, qualitatively different types of programs passed at different times within the same country can be used as negative cases for one another, as well as for different types of programs passed in different nations at the same time (see Orloff 1993). This is the strategy used in this book. Its use resulted in 19 cases for analysis: 4 for Canada, 7 for Australia, and 8 for the United States (see list in appendix A).

THE QUALITATIVE COMPARATIVE ANALYSIS

The QCA process begins with gathering the necessary information to identify suitable cases for comparison and specify case outcomes. The material gathered for these steps on the three nations in this work was included in the three preceding chapters; details of the process by which cases and outcome types were specified may be found in appendices A and B.

Once cases and outcomes have been specified, more detailed information on each factor must be gathered for each case and the pertinent information for analysis summarized in a specialized form of table, known as a "truth table." These steps can be made much less time consuming if the limited number of factors to be used in the QCA are chosen before the data is gathered. However, this shortened process assumes that the pertinent factors for analysis are already known, a presumption that may well limit research results to those that have produced several decades of theoretical confusion on this and other research questions.

This work took a different approach, which the author offers as an improvement to the commonly accepted methods of selecting independent variables for QCA (Amenta and & Poulsen 1994), especially on topics where conflicting research results predominate. This approach is to first gather data on all the potentially pertinent factors and then let the factors for inclusion in the QCA emerge from patterns in the data. (For details, see appendix C).

Once a truth table is constructed, mathematical techniques based on Boolean, or base two, algebra are used to analyze the information in the table. Essentially, the process uses Boolean algebra to express all the various combinations of causal factors that empirically precede a particular outcome and then to logically eliminate the factors irrelevant to that outcome (Ragin 1987). The result is a minimal expression of causation for a specific outcome.

As with quantitative systematic methods, the results of QCA are based on the association of causal factors with specific outcomes. The particular role of each such factor to each case can often be readily traced in the narrative of each nation's policy history. However, some factors may be directly related to outcomes without that relation being apparent in a policy narrative; such "behind-the-scenes" factors may create conditions conducive to policy successes without appearing to contribute to them in any obvious way. Several such conditions appear theoretically relevant to this research question and were included in the analysis.

In this book, data was gathered on 29 variables, which were later reduced to 16. (See appendices C and D for details.) Five outcome types were defined and clustered into two outcomes for the analysis, with NHI failure (F) as the negative type for NHI success (S). NHI failure was defined to include (1) "residual" programs, available only to the poor; (2) "dualistic" policies, which add public insurance for some categories of citizens and private insurance subsidies for the middle classes to residual programs; and (3) "universal dualistic" programs, which provide public insurance to all citizens, but at two different levels, depending on both market and nonmarket criteria. The first two are strictly market-based and do not appear to help build a legacy of universal health security; the third has recently appeared as a fallback position for anti-NHI forces in these nations, with unclear implications for the future. NHI success was defined to include (1) "partial" programs, with either some public health insurance for everyone or comprehensive insurance for most citizens, and (2) "decommodifying" programs, which provide comprehensive public insurance for all citizens. (For more details, see appendix B).

Examination of the summary data on these nineteen cases revealed four factors with the data pattern expected for necessary causal factors (present in all successful cases) and two with the data pattern expected for sufficient causal factors (absent in all cases resulting in failure). These six factors became the strongest candidates for inclusion in systematic analysis, and because of their high number in relation to the number of cases, effectively precluded the inclusion in the QCA of any additional factors. However, QCA using these six factors proved workable in spite of the relatively low number of cases. The results suggest that these four factors are necessary for NHI legislation to succeed in these nations: federal power in the health care area, a multiparty system, a legislative legacy, and strong trade unions (referred to hereafter as the "necessary" conditions). In addition, the analysis suggests that one of two interchangeable factors must be present in these nations for NHI success: a lack of veto points or labor party power (referred to hereafter as the "sufficient" conditions). These results were obtained as follows.

The truth table for these six variables is large and unwieldy, with sixty-four rows and eight columns (see appendix F). Empirical outcomes are found for only ten of the sixty-four possible configurations, placing concrete limits on the generalizability of the results.[3]

The presence of so many missing configurations in the truth table is an analytical problem, necessitating the use of specific methodological strategies. Three such strategies are available at this time for this method; each of these assigns outcomes to missing configurations in a different way, based on specific assumptions. These strategies allow flexibility in analysis, giving the researcher both conservative and more speculative approaches with which to establish the range of theoretical results compatible with the data. The approaches are: (1) the assignment of all missing configurations to a negative outcome; (2) the assignment of all such configurations to a positive outcome; and (3) the selective assignment of outcomes to all missing configurations on the basis of theoretical criteria. The third of these strategies proved useless in this analysis because of the large proportion of possible configurations not found in the data set; specifically, it resulted in conclusions identical to the criteria used to assign outcomes.[4] Useful analysis of this truth table was therefore limited to the first two approaches.

The first strategy, assigning all not-found configurations a negative outcome (F), amounts to the more conservative approach, in that the only configurations analyzed with outcome S are those so assigned through case data. The second strategy is therefore the more speculative approach and is mainly useful for learning the most reduced expression for S compatible with the data. Together, they establish the range of possible results compatible with the data.

Analysis of configurations with outcome S using the first, more conservative strategy produced the simplified expression S = BHJPQ +
BDHJQ, indicating that when NHI success has occurred in these nations,
a combination of factors has been present in one of two configurations.
(See appendix E for an introduction to Boolean language.) Specifically, the
four factors represented by the letters B, H, J, and Q have all been present; in addition, either the factor represented by the letter P or the factor
represented by the letter D has been present in all cases of NHI success.
The four ("necessary") conditions represented by these letters are federal
authority or leverage in the health area (B), a legislative health care legacy
(J), a multiparty system (H), and strong trade unions (Q); the two additional, interchangeable ("sufficient") conditions are a lack of veto points
(D) and labor party power (P).

That is, there are no cases with outcome S (NHI success) that do not
include all four necessary factors. However, two cases with outcome F
(NHI failure) exhibit the four necessary conditions with neither of the sufficient ones, so those four conditions are clearly insufficient to bring about
a successful NHI outcome by themselves. Similarly, all cases with either of
the sufficient factors present show outcome S; however, there are no cases
exhibiting either of the sufficient conditions that do not also show the
presence of the four necessary conditions.

The simplified expression S = BHJPQ + BDHJQ therefore
describes two overlapping configurations of conditions that have produced NHI victories in these nations. They are (1) a government in which
a labor party holds power (P), in a nation with a multiparty system, strong
trade unions, a legacy of state/provincial or federal health policy, and federal authority or financial leverage in the health area (the Australian
model) and (2) a nation with no veto points (D), a multiparty system,
strong trade unions, a legacy of state/provincial or federal health policy,
and federal authority or financial leverage in the health area (the Canadian model). The two models merge in Canada's third case, where no veto
points (D) and a labor party with power (P) were both present. There are
no cases with a successful NHI outcome that does not exhibit one of these
two configurations.

Both the models of NHI success for these nations also necessarily
include the "constants" identified previously for these nations (see appendix C): no other more decommodifying federal welfare state policy, a legacy
of public ownership and public subsidy of hospitals, politically organized
businesses, politically active trade unions, and politically organized medical

doctors. The findings above must therefore be considered limited to nations that share these conditions, which tend to institutionally legitimate government involvement in hospitals but not decommodifying welfare state policy and include both politically organized class-based supporters and opponents of NHI, plus one organized opposing interest group.

The result for S using the more speculative strategy is compatible with a far more limited set of causal conditions. When all not-found configurations are assigned positive outcomes, the result is S = D + P. The causal role of both the two sufficient variables (D, P) is therefore supported, but not the causal role of the four necessary conditions (B, H, J, P). This result casts some doubt on the role of these four factors in NHI success in these nations. However, the plausibility of this finding is more limited because the assumptions utilized in this strategy, that all missing configurations could occur and would always lead to NHI success, are so highly speculative.[5] This finding is therefore most useful for establishing the boundaries of the range of conclusions compatible with the data, which extends at its most extreme to the possibility that none of the four necessary conditions are necessary at all.

Analyses of the configurations for outcome (F) were also conducted but added nothing to the above results. Finally, the necessary and sufficient variables were checked separately to see whether those analyses could shed any further light on the findings (1) that outcome S requires the presence of either variable P or D, the sufficient variables, and (2) that outcome S also requires the simultaneous presence of variables B, H, J and Q, the necessary variables. More comprehensive testing is often possible in Boolean analysis with fewer variables, because a reduction in variables also reduces the proportion of missing to found configurations. The results supported the finding that one of the sufficient variables is necessary to produce S and showed that the variety of configurations exhibited by the nations in this study is not sufficient to determine definitively whether the necessary variables must also be present to produce S. (The interested reader will find the truth tables for these analyses in appendix F.)

The final step in the data analysis process was to address the data by nation. This analysis addressed the differences between NHI success and failure in each nation and contrasted the patterns of success for Canada and Australia with the closest pattern achieved by the United States. (See Summary Table by Nation in appendix F.) The results were as follows.

CANADA. Analysis of NHI failure and success in Canada shows that the difference between these two outcomes is institutional; the flexibility of Canada's institutions has allowed its sole constitutional veto point to be circumvented, strong unions developed, a successful legislative legacy built, and political power acquired by a minority labor party. Since labor party power developed only after the first NHI success in Canada, it is logically not necessary to the Canadian model of NHI success. However, national medical insurance and decommodifying NHI policy were notably introduced only after Canada's labor party became effective at the national level.

Canada exhibits only one negative case, its first. That case, and Canada's model of NHI failure, includes five negatives out of the six critical factors, with the only positive factor its multiparty system. Between that case and its second, successful case, Canada developed a legacy of provincial health insurance schemes and a strong trade union movement; even more important, it developed a tradition of regular federal-provincial negotiations and a legacy of federal financial subsidy of provincial health arrangements, circumventing its only veto point.

Canada's model of NHI success shows two configurations. In its second and fourth cases, Canada experienced successful NHI outcomes with a configuration of variables that included all four of the necessary conditions plus a lack of veto points. Its third case exhibits all these conditions plus labor party power, in this case the leverage of a parliamentary minority party. The main difference between NHI failure and success in Canada was, therefore, the circumvention of Canada's single constitutional veto point in response to social democratic and other electoral pressures, resulting in political institutional changes favorable to the passage of NHI.

An even more complete picture of Canada's model of NHI success can be developed by taking note of a few more factors. Within these three nations, Canada's historical legacy of public hospital management is unique, as are the constancy of executive and legislative majorities from the same political party. Furthermore, between Canada's negative and positive outcome cases, a federal health bureaucracy was developed. A legacy of public hospital management, same-party executives and legislative majorities, and the presence of a federal health bureaucracy are therefore also of possible importance in the Canadian model of NHI policy causation.

AUSTRALIA. Analysis of the Australian cases shows that the difference between failed and successful NHI outcomes in Australia has been Labor Party power. As in Canada, institutional changes were necessary to enable federal action; however, this was done in Australia through a national referendum to amend the constitution, sponsored and achieved by a Labor government in spite of active non-Labor opposition. In further contrast to Canada, Australian non-Labor governments have reversed NHI policies whenever elected, and the election of a Labor government has then been necessary for NHI's reinstatement. The tendency of non-Labor governments to move closer to Labor policy on health policy provisions over the past fifty years does not contradict this finding; it simply attests to the Labor policy's success and popularity.

Australia's four negative cases exhibit two different configurations, which differ only over federal power in the health field. That is, in Australia's first negative case, all the necessary factors were present except federal authority to act; in the next three, all four necessary factors are present. The Australian model for NHI failure therefore exhibits many more pro-NHI institutional variables than Canada's, reflecting Australian labor's early organizing and legislative successes at the state level; however, these were insufficient for NHI success even after federal authority to act was achieved.

Australia's three successful cases show only one configuration, which includes the four necessary conditions plus labor party power. Although the constitutional veto point for NHI was overcome in Australia, a second potential veto point remains, that of its second legislative body, the Senate; although a constitutional remedy is provided for such vetoes, that remedy depends upon the government's calling and winning a new election. So while veto points appear logically irrelevant to Australia's model of NHI success, that irrelevance actually depends on the Labor Party's power at the polls.

Australia also exhibits some relevant conditions not present in the other nations of this study, which cannot be tested systematically due to case limitations but may be of importance in the Australian model. These factors are state corporatism, preferential voting, and proportional representation, all of which are theorized to be conducive to NHI.

THE UNITED STATES. The United States' eight cases exhibit four configurations, all ending in NHI policy failure; there are therefore four U.S. models of NHI failure and no U.S. model of NHI success. All four of the U.S. configurations include the positive factor of federal authority in the health field and the negative factors of no multiparty system, multiple effective veto points, and no labor party power. The U.S. model of

NHI failure therefore exhibits a lack of both political institutional and class power factors. Analytically, NHI failed in the United States because it never achieved all of the necessary causal conditions at the same time or either of the two sufficient causal factors at any time.

This pattern can be further specified by examining the U.S. cases over time. Its first case shows the presence of only one of the necessary conditions, federal authority in the health care field. By the second case, strong trade unions were also present. However, by the third case in 1960, trade union strength had ebbed below the 30 percent benchmark, and no new positive factors appear. The fourth, fifth, and sixth cases show the largest number of positive factors for NHI exhibited for the United States; all are positive for trade union strength and a legislative legacy, as well as for federal authority. In the last two cases, however, union strength has again ebbed, with no new positive factors emerging. The first four U.S. cases mimic the phenomena seen in Canada and Australia of a buildup over time of conditions conducive to NHI, punctuated by periodic reversals in one factor. The final four U.S. cases contrast with those of Canada and Australia by exhibiting a pattern of failure to move forward on the other critical factors, followed by a decline in those necessary conditions that had already been achieved.

This analysis suggests that there may have been a critical window of opportunity for NHI in the United States between 1960 and 1975, when three of the four necessary factors were present there. The failure to achieve the fourth necessary factor, a multiparty system, before trade union strength went into long-term decline in the 1970s appears to have been critical to subsequent U.S. NHI failures. Progress during that time toward a national labor party, of course, might well have helped create a U.S. multiparty system and prevented a decline in union strength. It is also possible that a strong third-party effort to improve government in the United States by reducing or eliminating political veto points might have led to the same effects.

Notably, the U.S. pattern exhibits no unique conditions theorized as conducive to the passage of NHI. Instead, the United States exhibits three unique, theoretically negative factors: the lack of a multiparty political system, the absence of labor party power, and the presence of multiple veto points. Since all three of these factors were found to be either necessary or sufficient for the passage of NHI in these nations, all must be considered relevant to the failure of NHI in the United States.

RESULTS

The analysis has two principal findings. It strongly supports the finding that one of two sufficient conditions, a lack of veto points or labor party power, must be present in these three nations for NHI policy successes to occur. It somewhat less strongly supports the finding that four necessary conditions must also be present for NHI success: federal power in the health care area, a multiparty system, a legislative legacy, and strong trade unions. Taken separately or together, these findings suggest that in these nations, both political institutional and class power factors are relevant to the determination of national health policy.

While the limited number of cases in these nations prevents us from specifying the exact nature of this relevance, by looking at the above findings separately and then together, we can narrow the range of possibilities. That is, if only the first finding is correct, and either a lack of veto points or labor party power are sufficient to bring about NHI successes in these nations, then health policy can be determined either institutionally or social democratically, a finding of the type Ragin calls "multiple independent causation" (1987). In the unlikely case that the second finding alone is correct, health policy is determined by interaction between political institutional and class power factors; this would be the dynamic Ragin calls "conjunctural causation."

However, if both findings are correct, they suggest a more complex causal dynamic than Ragin specifies, requiring a fourth category to be added to the table of possible causal dynamics presented in the introduction to this book. That is, besides the possibility of (1) a single cause, (2) multiple independent causation, and (3) conjunctural causation, these results suggest a fourth model of causation. In that fourth model, conjunctural causation is present but occurs in more than one form. I call this dynamic "multiple conjunctural causation."[6]

Knowledge of this causal dynamic is important, in that it would present several puzzling features to researchers not methodologically equipped to consider a sufficient range of factors or prepared to test for such combinations of factors. That is, if causes can be both present and absent in cases leading and not leading to the outcome of interest, and the patterns unique to such dynamics are not known to researchers, as well as methods for identifying them, all such causes may appear to be irrelevant to the outcome of interest and falsely rejected for that reason. Specific research

TABLE 2.
MILLS' AND RAGIN'S MODELS OF CAUSATION EXPANDED

Patterns of Causation:	Method of Agreement: Is the causal factor present in all positive cases?	Indirect Method of Difference: Is the causal factor absent from all negative cases?
Single Causation: (one necessary and sufficient factor)	yes	yes
Multiple Independent Causation: (multiple sufficient but not necessary factors, interchangeable in their effect)	no	yes
Conjunctural Causation: (multiple necessary but not sufficient factors, causal in combination)	yes	no
Multiple Conjunctural Causation: (both of the preceding two patterns present; more than one form of conjunctural causation)	no	no

findings would then depend entirely on the specific subset of factors and cases considered. Such limitations could explain much of the contradictory and confusing findings in the literature on this research question.

In delineating this multiple conjunctural model of causation, this study has specified two paths to NHI policy success and one to NHI failure in these nations. Both the Canadian and Australian paths to NHI success exhibit one necessary class power resource and three necessary political institutional factors: strong trade unions, the development of federal authority or financial leverage in the health field, a multiparty system, and a legislative legacy in the health care field. In addition, both nations required one additional factor for success; however, in Canada that factor was institutional, while in Australia that factor was social democratic. Canada's path to NHI success therefore can be characterized as more institutional than Australia's, based on political flexibility around veto points, even though this occurred as a form of conservative compromise in the face of a growing labor party challenge. Australia's path to NHI success can be characterized as more social democratic than Canada's, based on a national Labor Party successfully overcoming veto points in the face of uncompromising non-Labor opposition through the mobilization of electoral support. In both nations, however, Labor party power and the ability to circumvent veto points only developed with the last of the four necessary conditions already specified. These paths therefore appear to exhibit interaction between both the necessary and sufficient causal factors and the political institutional and class power causal conditions.

The United States' path to NHI failure, in contrast, shows no cases including three of those conditions, two of which are political institutional and one social democratic. The United States has never developed a multiparty political system, a necessary institutional factor in Canada and Australia, and never developed either of the sufficient power resource or institutional factors for those nations, labor party power or circumvention of its veto points. The failure of NHI in the United States is therefore most fairly characterized from the evidence in this study as both political institutional and social democratic in form, and the evidence appears strong that the two are related.

Limitations and Generalization

As always, the results of a study must be considered limited by the range of cases examined. In this study, the results are clearly relevant only to these three nations on this type of modern policy question and can be generalized at most to nations that are culturally and institutionally similar to them. By this, I mean English-founded urbanized and industrialized capitalist democracies, which are also predominantly Protestant federations with divided political powers, similar demographics, dualistic economies, liberal welfare states, and a relatively high level of affluence.

In addition, these results must be considered limited to nations exhibiting the theoretically pro-NHI and anti-NHI conditions identified as "constants" for all the cases in these three nations. Those included a legacy of publicly owned hospitals, a legacy of public subsidy of hospitals, the presence of politically active trade unions, the absence of any other more decommodifying federal policies, the presence of politically organized business lobbies, and the presence of politically organized physicians.

The complexity of the findings, however, is quite likely to be representative of causal dynamics on modern policies in other types of nations and should serve as an object lesson to researchers using methods that can yield only simpler answers. The range of possibility of causal dynamics for such research questions must now be considered to include multiple variables and more than one causal model. Research that limits itself to fewer variables and simpler causal models is likely to lead only to more published studies with conflicting results and a lack of collective scientific progress on such questions.

CHAPTER 6

Conclusions

Two forms of comparative historical research were used in this book to address the question of U.S. exceptionality in national health policy. The results of the traditional analyses were reported at the end of the chapters on each nation's health politics and policies. Those findings, briefly stated, were as follows.

THEORETICAL CONCLUSIONS FROM THE TRADITIONAL STUDY

Canada

Canadian "Medicare" is actually a federally subsidized and coordinated system of provincial programs, characterized by its bipartisan support, popularity, and stability. Publicly assured access to health care in Canada became an issue in the western provinces around the turn of the century. As an area, health was constitutionally reserved in Canada to the provinces, but most of the power to tax was reserved to the federal government, making action difficult at either level of government. The first public health insurance program was created in the province of Saskatchewan under a socialist CCF government in 1946 and limited to hospitalization. After a few larger provinces also established limited public health insurance programs, a Liberal commonwealth government acted on a long-standing party promise by creating a federal program to subsidize provincial hospital insurance programs. This approach proved both workable and popular.

Once those subsidies began in 1958, another Saskatchewan CCF government introduced the first provincial medical insurance program, enduring a bitter doctor's strike in the process. A few years later, a Conservative-appointed royal commission, to everyone's surprise, recommended the adoption of public medical insurance across Canada along the lines of Saskatchewan's program. With the CCF/NDP (labor) party pressuring the Liberal government from the swing position in Parliament, that government proposed a federal subsidy for provincial medical insurance programs that met five basic criteria. The necessary legislation was passed in 1966, and all ten provinces had acted to join this program by 1971. Public control of medical costs and federal authority to require uniform conditions across Canada remained issues until 1984, when the program was strengthened on a unanimous parliamentary vote.

Canada's path to NHI, then, calls attention to its constitutional division of powers between the provinces and the commonwealth, the survival and growth of a socialist third party, the policy legacy pioneered by that party in a single minor province, and the relative lack of veto points to alter or block a Canadian government's legislative program under its parliamentary system. Canada's history also shows that vehement medical opposition to public health insurance has not been unique to the United States and that such opposition has not prevented the adoption of such programs elsewhere.

Australia

Public health insurance in Australia has been characterized by two politically polarized forms, major policy shifts with every change in government, and an evolving health policy legacy. Australia is the only industrialized democracy to have both instituted and dismantled a system of national health insurance, and it has done this twice.

Australia's political struggles over public health insurance began at about the same time as Canada's, with free hospitalization a labor issue in the state of New South Wales by 1908. Also as in Canada, action in the health field was constitutionally reserved to the states. Notably, this was not made an issue for the first national program passed there in 1938; sponsored by a non-Labor government, this program was compulsory and limited to low-income workers. However, because of medical opposition and the onset of World War II, this act was never implemented. A wartime Australian Labor government then introduced a free hospitalization program through the federal subsidy of state schemes and succeeded in getting a constitutional referendum passed authorizing federal action in the medical field. While this government's medical insurance program was never implemented because of medical noncooperation, its "free hospital experiment" lasted until 1952, when it was replaced by a non-Labor program with means-tested services for pensioners and benefits for the privately insured. However, even these limited programs soon created conflict between the state governments and organized medicine over costs.

Between 1972 and 1975, a Labor government reintroduced free hospitalization and proposed a medical federal insurance program called "Medibank"; when the non-Labor–dominated Senate refused to ratify Medibank, special constitutional provisions were invoked to break the deadlock, and Medibank was passed in a joint legislative session. However, the controversy cost Labor the next election, and both its free hospitalization and Medibank programs were phased out over the next six years, while non-Labor's means-tested pensioner program and private insurance subsidies were reinstated.

In 1983, a Labor government was elected, which reintroduced free hospitalization and its federal medical insurance program, renamed Medicare. The non-Labor government elected in 1996 then reintroduced a means-tested two-tiered system with one new, important feature; it places a majority of Australian citizens in the same category as pensioners and the poor, with the same higher level of public insurance. This appears to represent a significant compromise from previous non-Labor positions, in that it guarantees comprehensive health care coverage for most Australians likely to need it.

Australia's path to NHI calls attention to the role of its powerful Labor party, that party's successes using constitutional provisions to overcome political veto points and the legacy of health care protection built up there over time in spite of medical noncooperation and the repeated dismantling of NHI programs by non-Labor governments. Like Canada, Australia experienced determined opposition by organized medicine, but that opposition was not successful in permanently blocking NHI.

The United States

Efforts to assure access to health services in the United States also began at the state level around the turn of the century. By 1913, a nationally coordinated campaign had been organized to pass state programs for compulsory health insurance for industrial workers and their dependents. Opposition by the AMA, and the nation's entrance into World War I, effectively ended this campaign. However, in contrast to Canada and Australia, the U.S. government's authority to act in the health field was not a constitutional issue.

A federally subsidized, state-based medical program was considered by President Roosevelt as part of the Social Security Bill of 1935 but abandoned because of organized medical opposition; a similar 1939 effort led by legislators was killed in committee, as were more limited bills in 1941, 1943, and 1944. President Truman made strong efforts to get universal, comprehensive national medical insurance passed between 1945 and 1949; he was defeated by a combination of AMA opposition and targeting by the anti-Communist extremists who came to dominate congressional politics during that time.

National health insurance was so thoroughly defeated in the United States by 1950 that no more efforts to introduce it were made until 1958, and then they were limited to hospitalization insurance for the aged. This legislator-led proposal generated such public support, however, that a powerful congressional Democratic opponent of the bill was moved to sponsor a more limited bill in 1960, resulting in the Kerr-Mills program of federally subsidized state insurance programs for the elderly poor. President Kennedy revived the proposal of national hospitalization insurance for all the elderly in 1961; however, that bill was blocked in legislative committee until after the 1965 "landslide" Democratic victory under President Johnson. Even then, concessions to organized medicine and the bill's conservative opponents were necessary; a federally subsidized private medical insurance option was added to Medicare, and the Kerr-Mills program was expanded into Medicaid, a subsidized state insurance program for the poor.

No pro-NHI initiatives have succeeded in the United States since 1965. Efforts by President Nixon and legislative health care advocates in the 1970s to address both escalating costs and care inequities failed when all the supporters needed were unable to agree on a compromise bill. In 1993, President Clinton initiated a major effort to pass national health insurance; however, conservative opposition, committee delaying tactics, and the introduction of several competing bills prevented either house from even taking a floor vote on NHI. The means-tested State Children's Health Insurance Program, adopted in 1997, represents more of a shift in the use of Medicaid funds than a step toward NHI. It and the 2003 Medicare Prescription Drug Act appear to trade off the privatization of publicly financed services for small increases in citizen access or financial protection.

NHI dynamics in the United States draw attention to divisions over health policy within the Democratic Party, the presence of multiple political veto points with no constitutionally provided remedies, and the resultant success of NHI's opponents in blocking comprehensive legislation and shaping more limited proposals. When compared to Canada and Australia, these dynamics call particular attention to the U.S. federal division of powers, its lack of a national labor party, and the heightened influence on U.S. policy of organized groups like the AMA.

The differences between the three nations in national health policy therefore appear to reflect the nations' differences on a coherent set of political institutional and power resource causal factors. These include the constitutional and institutional division of federal and subfederal powers creating effective veto points for policy, the presence or absence of an effective labor party, and the health policy legacy created over time at both the subfederal and federal levels of government. These factors appear to operate in conjunction with one another, or interactively. Contrary to U.S. popular thinking, AMA opposition by itself cannot explain U.S. exceptionalism on this issue, because equally strong and determined medical interest groups were present but unable to dominate policymaking in both Canada and Australia.

WHAT THE SYSTEMATIC STUDY ADDS

The systematic analysis reported in chapter 5 supports the finding of the traditional historical analyses that NHI policy successes and failures in Australia, Canada, and the United States were determined by political institutional and class power factors. In addition, this study identifies more specific sets of causal conditions that act in conjunction with one another in these nations, including two causal factors not identified by the traditional analysis. The systematic study therefore adds to the traditional analysis by further specifying its findings and by more precisely relating them to NHI outcomes in Canada, Australia, and the United States.

The qualitative comparative analysis (QCA) found four necessary conditions that must be present simultaneously for NHI policy successes to occur in these nations. Three of those are political institutional factors: federal authority or financial leverage in the health field, a multiparty system, and a legislative legacy. The fourth is a power resource factor: strong trade unions. In addition, the QCA found that one of two sufficient factors must be present for NHI successes, neither of which developed in any of these nations before the four necessary conditions. One of the two sufficient factors, a lack of veto points, is political institutional; the other, labor party power, is social democratic. The QCA found no NHI successes in any of these nations without the presence of all four of the necessary factors, plus one of these two sufficient conditions.

The central role of four of these factors was made fairly clear by the traditional analysis; the importance of federal authority or financial leverage, a lack of veto points, labor party power, and a health policy legacy were all strongly suggested there. However, the two additional causal factors identified by the systematic study, a multiparty system and strong trade unions, were not identified by the traditional analysis because of its less deliberate use of measures. That is, few of the sources on this question focus directly on either of these factors or compare them in times of NHI success and failure, making them easy to overlook. However, the relevance of both factors was suggested in the theoretical literature on this question, so specific, comparable information was sought on them for the more systematic QCA. As a part of that process, criteria were created to distinguish multiparty systems from two-party systems in these nations, and strong trade union movements from weak ones. The results were then entered into case summary tables, resulting in the ready identification of the two factors as closely correlated with NHI outcomes and worthy of further analysis, along with the other four necessary and sufficient factors.

The QCA then specified the Canadian and Australian paths to NHI in terms of the six necessary and sufficient factors. The Canadian path exhibits one class power and four political institutional factors, including a lack of veto points; it is compatible with the theoretical explanation of NHI success as the result of adaptive political institutional responses to popular demand, including social democratic organization. The Australian path exhibits three political institutional and two power resource factors; its NHI successes fit the theoretical explanation of working-class organization leading to political power and the ability to force changes in both political institutions and national policy. The United States, in contrast, has never developed two of the critical institutional factors or one of the critical class power factors identified: a multiparty system, a lack of veto points, or labor party power. Since one of those institutional factors, a multiparty system, preceded the development of either of the other two critical factors in Canada and Australia, the U.S. path can fairly be described as representing the institutional blockage of social democratic change.

These findings support the conclusion that national health policy in these nations is determined by the interaction of political institutional and power resource factors. This follows from two facts. The first is that the simultaneous presence of all the necessary and sufficient political institutional factors was not sufficient in these nations to allow the passage of NHI without the additional presence of a class power factor, strong trade unions. In addition, although NHI success did occur whenever both the necessary and sufficient power resource factors were present, both of these factors never occurred without three of the four critical political institutional factors. Since both models of NHI success in these nations require both political institutional and power resource factors in specific combinations, their effect is logically interactive rather than additive.[1]

SO WHAT?

Two specific findings for the United States are suggested by this work. The first is that U.S. exceptionalism in national health policy represents the institutional blockage of social democratic change. That is, neither the original constitutional arrangements nor the traditions developed in Congress have proven to be class neutral. Policy changes friendly to American workers have been disadvantaged by these institutional structures, which allow economically powerful minority interests to dominate the legislative process. This domination has resulted not only in perpetual vetoes of worker-friendly legislation but also in the reduction in number and scope of such initiatives and the production of highly compromised policy outcomes. In addition, the presence of so many veto points has rendered the system unaccountable; when no legislator need cast a public vote on such legislation, none can be held responsible by voters for failing to support it. As Maioni suggests, the supposedly ideals-based U.S. "aversion to government" may actually be the result of dissatisfaction with the American political experience and a consequence of America's unresponsive political institutions (1998:29).

The second finding suggested by this research is that both political institutional changes and social democratic organization may be necessary for the United States to achieve NHI success. If the United States follows the path taken by its most similar nations, Canada and Australia, NHI success will require (1) the development of a multiparty system and (2) the revival of strong trade unions, followed by either (3) the elimination or circumvention of our multiple political veto points or (4) the development of a labor party with some national power. Because Canada and Australia exhibit somewhat different models of NHI success, however, the findings also leave open the possibility that the United States may evolve its own unique political institutional and social democratic path to national health insurance. Both Canada and Australia's histories suggest that such evolution would be encouraged by state-level experimentation with universal public hospital insurance, especially if federal subsidies were provided.

More generally, this work's results suggest that welfare state policies are far more complex in their causation than generally theorized. Indeed, more than one of the theories put forward about such processes appear to be accurate under different historical and cultural conditions; the primary job of researchers may be the specification of the conditions under which each theory accurately describes policy dynamics. This study strongly suggests that in historically and culturally similar nations, a core group of necessary causal factors may be shared, but one of a set of sufficient causal conditions may also be required to bring about the outcome of interest. It leaves open the possibility that historically and culturally diverse nations may arrive at similar policy outcomes through very different causal paths.

Finally, the research results support the assertion that the very safeguards against tyranny built into the United States Constitution at this point support continuing or increasing U.S. economic inequality, by making it easy to block the social democratic route to decreasing that inequality. The multiple points at which majority governance may be thwarted appear to have created a dynamic where a discouraged majority allows a determined minority to rule. While such minority rule may occasionally grant concessions to well-organized and aggressively asserted majority pressure, it need not allow fundamental enough concessions or administer those concessions granted in such a way as to actually disrupt minority dominance.

While hardly a new assertion, this dynamic is worthy of further specification. For instance, the massive amounts of "red tape" in the United States attributed to the existence of too large a federal bureaucracy may logically be a product of the specific difficulties posed by the U.S. constitutional balance-of-powers arrangement. Arguably, these factors reduce the workability of American political processes, repeatedly forcing legislation into compromising contradictions. Complex details, exceptions, and contradictions logically slow government action and reduce its efficiency, providing ammunition with which to attack government action as inherently ineffective and inefficient. These factors then may feed mass discouragement with the voting process and its results, reducing participation in voting and further reducing the political effectiveness of the majority.

Therefore, the most important suggestion of this research for American democracy is that unless we make major changes to our political institutions, making them more responsive to citizen majorities, and our politicians more accountable for policy, we can expect more problems of the same sort. The organized minorities that presently dominate law and policy making in the United States are not likely to relinquish such power voluntarily, and as long as their domination perpetuates political inequality, bureaucratic inefficiency, and citizen discouragement, the problem will not correct itself. Problems capable of solution by responsive governments will remain perpetually unsolved in the United States, and many of the chief blessings of democracy will, ironically, elude those pioneers of democracy, the American people.

LIMITATIONS TO THE STUDY

As usual, there are limitations to this work and ambiguities in its results. One important set of factors could not be adequately examined. A central assumption in the study's design was the availability of sufficient secondary or primary data to allow all theoretically relevant factors to be systematically compared for the three nations. During the research process, it was found that much needed data on the unity or division of interests within relevant categories of politically organized actors had not been published and could not be obtained without extensive access to primary sources in all three nations. As a consequence, those factors had to be excluded from the systematic study.

In addition, the analysis remains somewhat incomplete due to methodological limitations. While a core set of political institutional and power resource factors was identified as causal to the policy of all three nations, some additional factors that may be important in the policy dynamics of the individual nations could not be confirmed or rejected, due to the limited number of factors that can presently be analyzed for such a limited number of cases. The finding of multiple conjunctural causation in this work suggests that social scientists have much more work to do before our understanding of empirical reality at the national level can approach mastery. Theoretically, we need more sophisticated models for complex interactive dynamics. Methodologically, our ability to test complex causal dynamics at the national level remains limited.

As usual, the theoretical approach and subsequent research design may have, in some measure, affected the study's results. For instance, this work has interpreted such factors as business lobbies and trade unions as class power resources rather than interest-group forces and interpreted the study's results through a social democratic prism. No systematic way is currently known to study and seek to understand such relationships without some such prism, and the potential errors inherent in that limitation must be acknowledged.

This study handled the problem of potential bias by gathering information on as many nontargeted factors as possible, in order to allow evidence of nontargeted causes to emerge in the data. In addition, the choice of variables for the systematic analysis was then made from patterns in the data, rather than from the researcher's favored explanation. The combined use of these precautions supports the validity of the findings. While labor intensive, and therefore rejected for practical reasons by many researchers, these analytical processes are offered as a way to minimize potential bias, improve the usefulness of research for testing multiple competing hypotheses, and improve our ability to understand complex causal processes.

DIRECTIONS FOR FUTURE RESEARCH

This book suggests some directions for future research. Similar studies of other welfare state issues, and of the same issues within other welfare state regimes, would be useful for discovering other causal dynamics, as well as testing the accuracy and generalizability of these findings. Comparative studies of the impacts of different types of policies, among "most dissimilar" as well as "most similar" nations, would be useful to illuminate the full range of possibilities for effective welfare state policy. It would be particularly useful to see cross-national research done on the types of national policy that lead to effective health care cost containment.

The methods used here would be useful for the exploration of past or present differences in state or provincial welfare state policies. The impact and interaction of each of the conditions determining health policies should be measured quantitatively, where possible, and new methodological techniques developed to allow testing of the additional causal factors suggested to be important for individual nations. Most important, since specifying all these dynamics will pit researchers squarely against the problem of multiple variables and relatively few cases, methodological innovation is critical to progress in this area.

In all three of the nations discussed in this book, primary research is needed on the unity or division of interests within the major categories of politically organized actors over time. In the United States, it would be very useful to have comparative studies of political institutional dynamics on welfare state issues in states where power is as divided as at the federal level and states in which fewer veto points exist. Both of these types of research would help clarify the effects of such dynamics on broad class-based initiatives and shed further light on the findings of this work.

The ability of social scientists to specify the causal mechanisms and dynamic processes of public policy appears to be steadily improving. It is hoped that this book will both add to our collective understanding of that area and encourage future progress in it.

Appendices

APPENDIX A

The Selection of Cases

Differences between U.S. political institutions and the parliamentary system used in Australia and Canada raised an important analytical issue for this research project: how to identify the appropriate time periods for cases in the United States. These periods were readily identified for Australia and Canada by the tenure of specific governments and their sponsorship of legislation relevant to NHI; under the parliamentary system, majority party sponsorship guarantees both executive support and a realistic chance of legislative action. However, because legislative majorities are unconnected in the United States with the choice of executive, there is no similar correlation there between majority party sponsorship, executive support, and legislative action.

For instance, legislative bills in the United States can be sent to Congress by the president and often are; however, such bills also require congressional sponsors, can be vastly altered without the president's permission, and face competing bills introduced by legislators without presidential approval. The passage of legislation then requires approval by potentially hostile legislative committees, which may choose to act or not act on specific bills; assignment by the majority leader to a hostile committee has been a frequent burial ground for legislation.

Even if the majority of a committee is favorably disposed toward a bill, a powerful committee chair can single-handedly block action, as Rep. Wilbur Mills did for four years to President Kennedy's, then President Johnson's, Medicare initiative. A hostile committee or chair can also amend a bill in such a way as to reverse its intended effects. If a bill is voted intact out of all its committees, it still faces inaction or hostile amendment on the floor of the House or Senate; the support of the majority leader is again essential to success at this point.

Conversely, Congress may initiate and pass a bill that is hostile to the president's policies. When this happens, the president can veto the bill, sending it back to Congress for further action or abandonment. However, a two-thirds majority of both houses can overrule a presidential veto.

Even when the president and legislative majorities are from the same political party, there is no necessary connection in the United States between executive support and a realistic chance of legislative action. Presidents who advocated health policy in their campaigns or legislative addresses, even with congressional majorities from their own political party, have frequently been unable to get their bills out of committee, much less to a floor vote. True "windows" for action are harder to identify than in Canada or Australia.

The designation of appropriate cases in the United States is further complicated by the staggered timing of executive and legislative elections. That is, U.S. presidents are elected on a four-year cycle and can only serve two terms, while representatives are elected every two years and senators every six years. Elections may therefore alter the legislative majority in either house several times during the tenure of any president, as may deaths, resignations, or party switching by individual legislators. Specific criteria were therefore needed to identify appropriate U.S. time periods for comparison to the Canadian and Australian cases.

This problem was handled by the use of three criteria, all of which must be met for period inclusion. These were as follows:(1) public presidential promotion of legislation that promotes health care financing arrangements that are more public and less commodified than those in place at the time; (2) presidential sponsorship or endorsement of a specific such bill that is introduced in Congress; and (3) senior sponsors from the majority party and the announced support of the majority leadership for such legislation in both houses of Congress.

These criteria presume that presidential support is a practical necessity for such controversial legislation to pass in the United States, because the two-thirds majority vote necessary to overrule a presidential veto is relatively difficult to achieve and because presidents are in an excellent position to mobilize public and legislative support or opposition (Fein 1986:135; Hage and Hollingsworth 1995). Second, these criteria assume that public presidential support for a popular issue such as NHI, combined with failure to send a bill to Congress, shows either a lack of real commitment to that issue or a negative assessment of such an initiative's chance of legislative action. Third, these criteria recognize that legislation has no chance of passage without influential majority party support in both houses of Congress.

What these criteria do not address is the difficult problem of hidden or unrecorded presidential and legislative dynamics; no systematic way is known to sort out these dynamics using available records. In addition, these criteria do not address the difficult issue of party and ideological differences over program design, particularly those of primarily private, minimal approaches versus primarily public, decommodifying approaches. It is certainly easiest to pass legislation if the president and a majority of both houses of Congress agree on such an approach, but it is an empirical question whether such agreement must exist before the legislative process begins or can be created during the process.

These processes resulted in the delineation of nineteen cases, described as negative or positive by the criteria detailed in the next appendix. The letter and number that follow each case in parentheses (C1, U8) are the sequential case designations used in the tables.

1. Canada, 1945. Negative Case. (C1)
2. Canada, 1955–57. Positive Case. (C2)
3. Canada, 1963–71. Positive Case. (C3)
4. Canada, 1980–84. Positive Case. (C4)
5. Australia, 1938. Negative Case. (A1)
6. Australia, 1941–49. Positive Case. (A2)
7. Australia, 1950–72. Negative Case. (A3)
8. Australia, 1972–75. Positive Case. (A4)
9. Australia, 1975–83. Negative Case. (A5)
10. Australia, 1983–96. Positive Case. (A6)
11. Australia, 1996–2000. Negative Case. (A7)
12. United States, 1934–44. Negative Case. (U1)
13. United States, 1946–49. Negative Case. (U2)
14. United States, 1960. Negative Case. (U3)
15. United States, 1961–64. Negative Case. (U4)
16. United States, 1965. Negative Case. (U5)
17. United States, 1969–76. Negative Case. (U6)
18. United States, 1993–94. Negative Case. (U7)
19. United States, 1995–2000. Negative Case. (U8)

APPENDIX B

A Typology of Health Policy Outcomes

The qualities of interest gathered to typify program outcomes initially included amounts and types of state involvement, the inclusion or exclusion of private insurance companies, the categories of citizens covered, the comprehensiveness of health care coverage, separate or identical health care arrangements for those relying on public insurance, the allowance or prohibition of patient co-payments, the allowance or prohibition of higher than publicly "scheduled" physician fees, and program financing. As information on the methods of financing programs often proved to be less available than the other information, and program financing was frequently altered many times during a program's life, that data was not used in typifying case outcomes.

Those outcomes were then typed in a two-part process, beginning with the two characteristics used to identify NHI outcomes in this study, that is, whether each was decommodifying or public. The definition of those characteristics and their application to the cases in this study is described below. A second classification method, based on the variance in programs among these nations, was then applied to check the usefulness of the initial typology. On the basis of this second method, programs defined as "public" were split into three categories, enabling five policy outcome types to be delineated, two representing NHI successes and three, NHI failures.

For this study, policy was defined as *public* if it (1) mandated financial protections or health care services for citizens or (2) provided for significant public control over the arrangements that determine access to care and/or the financial impact of health care costs. For instance, governmental subsidy of market driven private insurance would not be considered public, but the subsidy of private insurance meeting public standards of availability and comprehensiveness would be considered public.

Policy was defined as *decommodifying* if it (1) removed market factors in citizen access to care or insurance and (2) removed market-based divisions in the quantity and quality of care available to citizens. Policy that made health insurance universal, rather than available through the workplace or market, would therefore be decommodifying, but policy that set up a separate system for those uninsured through the labor or insurance market would not.

The use of "or" and "and" statements with these criteria should be carefully noted. Policy was considered public if it met either of the two public criteria; in contrast, policy was only characterized as decommodifying if it met both of the decommodifying criteria. Decommodification was therefore conceptualized as the more demanding of the two characteristics and, as will be seen, has been the quality least likely to characterize health care policy in these three nations. For instance, U.S. Medicare and Australian non-Labor health policy satisfy the public criteria but do not meet the criteria for decommodification.

The criteria given above were defined as follows. For the public criteria, "mandates" meant compulsory rather than voluntary, and "financial protections" might be either public or private. "Health care services," for the purposes of this study, included medical and hospital services, which might be made available through financing provisions, regulation, public ownership and management, or public employment of service providers. "Significant public control" could be secured through regulation, ownership and management, or employment of service providers.

For the decommodifying criteria, "market factors" included all factors related to the labor and health care markets. Labor market factors included income, employment benefits, and any restriction of benefits to citizens in categories related to labor, such as employment status, disability, or old age. Health care market factors included such provisions to control the cost of health care as care provision arrangements, consumer information and alternatives, negotiated or contracted fees for services, and other budget controls. "Market-based divisions in the quantity and quality of care" are held to have been removed when the same health care options are made available to all citizens without regard to any market factors and without any indication to service providers of the insured's financial resources or relation to the labor market. In particular, the destruction of the private health care system is not seen as necessary to decommodify care, as long as that system has been made irrelevant to care access, quantity, and quality for most workers. Such irrelevance might be achieved by providing equivalent facilities, shrinking the private system, providing public access to that system, or other such mechanisms.

Four combinations of these two characteristics are logically possible, three of which were found in this study:

1. Type 0: neither public or decommodifying.
2. Type P: public but not decommodifying.

3. Type D: decommodifying but not public. (Not found.)
4. Type PD: public and decommodifying.

Programs that simply supplement voluntary market arrangements by insuring some of those unable to secure services through the market, such as U.S. Medicaid, or by supplementing voluntary insurance premiums, such as U.S. Medicare Part B, were categorized as Type 0 programs. Arrangements that provide for public insurance with significant public control, but available only to the elderly or disabled like U.S. Medicare Part A, would be Type P. Canadian Medicare and Australian Medicare under its Labor governments would be examples of Type PD programs, in that they are universal and provide for significant public control. There were no instances of Type D among these nations, because private programs in these three nations are market based, commodifying both health services and financial protection (insurance); although many of the medical facilities in these nations developed through private, charitable organizations that continue to supplement their work, none of the three nations evolved health care systems based on such organizations. Table 3 summarizes the typification of each case's outcome by the criteria given above.

The usefulness of these typologies was then checked using a second classification approach. The goal in creating a typology of health welfare states is to typify these programs in a reasonably simple, theoretically useful, and methodologically elegant way. The central problem in producing such a typology is the number of ways in which actual national policies vary, by (1) citizens covered, (2) services included, (3) different approaches to partial coverage of services, and (4) differences in all the preceding at a given point in time between a nation's subfederal units of government, in particular, the states or provinces.

I therefore constructed a table of policy types using the two most distinct of these variables (1) citizens covered and (2) services included, with categories constructed to fit (3) above, and to allow for the variance in (4) above. The cases were then entered into this table. The result, with one additional modification, was table 4.

All the case outcomes in the bottom row of this table, by definition, correspond to type 0; that is, such programs are neither public nor decommodifying in their effects. Examples include the U.S. Kerr-Mills program and pre-1996 Australian non-Labor programs. Furthermore, the top left cell of this table is the only one in which type PD programs appear, that

TABLE 3.
CASE TYPIFICATION BY OUTCOME: PUBLIC (P), DECOMMODIFYING (D)

	P1	*P2*	*P*	*D1*	*D2*	*D*	*Type*
C1*	-	-	-	-	-	-	(0)**
C2	-	+	+	-	-	-	P
C3	+	+/-	+	-	-	-	P
C4	+	+	+	+	+	+	PD
A1	-	-	-	-	-	-	(0)
A2	+	+/-	+	-	-	-	P
A3	+	-	+	-	-	-	P
A4	+	+/-	+	+	-	-	P
A5	+	-	+	-	-	-	P
A6	+	+	+	+	+	+	PD
A7	+	+	+	-	+	-	P
U1	-	-	-	-	-	-	(0)
U2	-	-	-	-	-	-	(0)
U3	-	-	-	-	-	-	0
U4	-	-	-	-	-	-	0
U5	+	-	+	-	-	-	P
U6	+	+/-	+	-	-	-	P
U7	+	+/-	+	-	-	-	P
U8	+	+/-	+	-	-	-	P

(+) = positive, (-) = negative, (+/-) = mixed results.

*The codes in the left-hand column refer to the sequentially numbered cases from each nation: A = Australia, C = Canada, U = United States.

**Types in parentheses indicate the main type of state or provincial policy in place before passage of national legislation.

is, programs that are public and decommodifying, such as Canadian Medicare after 1984 or Australian Medicare under Labor governments. In effect, then, all pro-NHI political struggles have as their objective moving national health policy from the bottom right-hand cell of this table to its upper left-hand cell, and all other cells of the table contain cases that represent either compromises or failures for pro-NHI forces.

Furthermore, the right-hand column holds all the cases that represent outright failures for pro-NHI forces or reversals in health policy by anti-NHI governments. Those in the four upper-left cells, on the other hand, all represent pro-NHI successes. I therefore attached numbers to all

TABLE 4.
CASE OUTCOME TYPES, CATEGORIZED BY CITIZENS
AND SERVICES COVERED

	Comprehensive public benefits	Public benefits vary by type (hospital, medical, etc.)	Public benefits supplement or support private market (dualistic)
Universal coverage	A6, C4 Type PD A4 Type P3 "decommodifying"	A2 Type P3 "partial"	A7 Type P2 "universal dualistic"
Dualistic coverage (varies by citizen category or market position)	C3 Type P3 "partial"	C2 Type P3 "partial"	A3, A5,U5, U6, U7, U8 Type P1 "dualistic"
Residual coverage (means-tested only)			U3, U4 Type 0 U1, U2, A1, C1 Type (0) "residual"

A = Australia, C = Canada, U = United States.
P = public, PD = public and decommodifying, 0 = neither.
Shading represents designation as NHI success (darker) or failure (lighter) in this study.
Types in parentheses indicate the main type of state or provincial policy in place before passage of national legislation.

the "P" category cases to distinguish between policy defeats for pro-NHI forces (resulting in policy types 0, P1 or P2) and policy successes (resulting in policy types P3 or PD). Examples of the first include Australian non-Labor programs and the compromise that resulted in U.S. Medicare. Examples of pro-NHI successes include the "free hospital experiment" in Australia and Canada's NHI policy changes since 1955. These observations support the usefulness of the P/PD typology, and provide evidence of its flexibility.[1]

The result was the following types:

1. (Type 0):   *Residual* programs: means-tested (available only to the poor; stigmatized).

2. (Type P1): *Dualistic* programs: restricted to qualifying categories, means-tested for the poor, supplemental for the privately insured.

3. (Type P2): *Universal Dualistic* programs: universal, but with two levels of coverage tied to market position for most citizens, plus subsidies for the privately insured.

4. (Type P3): *Partial* programs: limited or comprehensive public insurance offered to all citizens on an equal basis, with required fees limiting access for some citizens.

5. (Type PD): *Decommodifying* programs: comprehensive public insurance offered to all citizens, with no limitations on access based on the ability to pay fees.

These types form an ordinal progression in the political struggle over NHI in these nations. Residual programs offer the lowest level of protection to citizens of the four types; all three countries began the century with residual local or state/provincial programs, and the first national programs passed in two of the three nations were residual in type. Dualistic programs offer a somewhat higher level of protection to citizens than residual programs but separate access provisions for the poor and retirees from financial protections for the employed middle classes. Such programs have been the preference of NHI opponents in all three nations when forced to seriously consider passing a national health program, presumably because they create anti-NHI policy and market legacies.

Universal dualistic programs provide access to care and financial protections for most citizens but maintain some divisions in the quality or amount of care or protection by market position. They therefore offer better protections to most citizens than dualistic programs but appear more ideologically acceptable to NHI opponents than decommodifying programs. Such a program was found in only one case in these three nations, adopted by the current nonLabor Australian government as its alternative to Labor's successful decommodifying program. Universal dualistic programs therefore represent a new form of compromise in these nations, which may be chosen by NHI opponents when anything less than a universal national program would be politically problematic.

Partial programs are offered to all citizens on an equal basis, although real access may be restricted by some criteria or the ability to pay a partial fee. Such programs do not necessarily provide more protection for citizens than dualistic programs but appear to create a political legacy amenable to the adoption of more protective programs. The two nations in this book that passed partial programs later adopted decommodifying programs, which offer the highest level of access to care and financial protection of the four types.

It is therefore possible to fairly characterize residual or dualistic programs as representing defeats for pro-NHI forces in these nations and partial or decommodifying programs as NHI victories. Universal dualistic programs could be either, but the only case of such a program in these nations was adopted as an alternative to the decommodifying program in place so is properly characterized as an NHI defeat. This additional modification allows the typology to be reduced when necessary, as it was with the limited number of cases in this work, to a binary typology of NHI failure (F) or success (S). This consolidation of outcome types produced six positive and thirteen negative cases for systematic analysis.

APPENDIX C

The Choice of Causal Factors

Information was gathered for these cases on all the factors identified in the introduction as pertinent to these theories. Comparable information was obtained for twenty-nine variables. However, preliminary analysis made it clear that qualitative comparative analysis was unworkable with so many variables and so few cases.

A closer look at the analytic process clarified the limits on the numbers of usable variables relative to the number of cases. QCA utilizes configurations as the basic unit of analysis. A configuration is a unique combination of relevant conditions or factors, with each such factor defined as a dichotomous variable; two dichotomous conditions may combine in four possible ways (2^2), and three conditions produce eight possible configurations (2^3).

In sorting out the results of these causal combinations, it can be readily seen that it would be helpful to have at least one empirical case exhibiting each possible configuration in order to determine the relation of individual factors to outcomes. For instance, if both federal power and legislative legacies are found to be present in every case resulting in NHI, both are likely causal factors for that outcome. However, if there are no cases found in which one condition is present and the other absent, the possibility that only one of the two is necessary for that outcome cannot be logically eliminated.

The number of cases and their configurational variation is therefore closely related to the number of factors that can be systematically tested using QCA; ideally, the number of possible configurations should exceed the number of actual cases by as little as possible. By this reasoning, 19 cases is insufficient to systematically test more than 5 to 6 factors, which yield 32 (2^5) to 64 (2^6) possible configurations.

In this type of analysis, it is also helpful to specify outcomes in a limited number of ways, because the division of cases into more than two outcome types further reduces the number of empirical configurations available for each analysis, exacerbating the problem just described. For this study, therefore, types 0, P1, and P2 were merged into a category labeled "NHI failure" (F), and types P3 and PD were combined into a category labeled "NHI success" (S). A search of the literature revealed that most published studies using qualitative comparative analysis with a comparable number of cases have limited themselves to five factors and two types of outcomes (Hicks et al. 1995; Hicks 1994; Weinberg and Gould 1993; Ganguly 1997; Ragin et al. 1984).

The total number of variables for this study was initially reduced in two ways, (1) by identifying and setting aside factors that acted as constants in these cases and (2) by combining measures of theoretically similar variables that showed similar empirical results. Six factors were eliminated as constants in these cases and 7 by combining related factors, leaving 16 variables. (See list in appendix D.)

At this point, an appropriate process was sought for selecting the most appropriate factors for systematic analysis. Such a process would have to respect the logic of the chosen method, including both theoretical considerations and the integrity of the data. Those concerns led to an examination of the data for patterns, using Mills' methods of agreement and indirect difference. The reduced summary table was scrutinized for factors that were consistently positive in cases with a positive outcome (S) and factors that were consistently negative in cases with a negative outcome (F). Any condition exhibiting either pattern would be a strong candidate for causation. In addition, any factor exhibiting both patterns would meet the criteria for a single-factor explanation.

Two factors (D,P) showed consistently negative results in the cases with negative outcomes, and four (B,H,J,Q) exhibited consistently positive results in the cases with positive outcomes. No factors showed both patterns. These observations can be verified in table 5.

These 6 factors constituted a reasonably manageable number for systematic analysis using 19 variables. Before proceeding further with this set of factors, however, their theoretical and methodological suitability for this study was evaluated. As variables emerging from patterns in the data, their theoretical relevance was not a concern. Methodologically, the most important consideration in the selection of causal factors for analysis is whether any of the excluded measures might logically lead to other research conclusions.

Nine of the 10 excluded factors were noted to exhibit 3 specific patterns. The first is more specific to nation than to outcome, and the second is more sensitive to time than to outcome. The third pattern combines a time element with the reappearance of an earlier condition and appears more likely to result from NHI outcomes then to help determine them. Since these excluded measures appear more related to specific nations, to time, or to the results of NHI outcomes than to its determination, none of them appears to offer much additional comparative explanatory power. Their inclusion is therefore unlikely to produce different results than analysis of the 6 factors alone, although they may be important to understanding the dynamics of specific nations or of the overall process.

There is, however, one measure that shows no particular pattern; executive and legislative majorities from the same political party (E) exhibits positive results in all except four cases, with mixed outcomes. This political institutional measure was primarily included to consider its mitigating effect on veto points; however, although in many cases it is observed to be positive when the measure of veto points is negative, the outcomes are too mixed for any such effect to be apparent. Some relation between this variable and the outcome of interest cannot be ruled out, although it appears a weaker causal candidate than the six emergent factors; however, it could not be tested with the six emergent factors within the limits of this data. Fortunately, because this factor is political institutional, like four of the six emergent variables, empirical support for it would appear unlikely to change the essential theoretical findings of the study.

The six factors emerging from patterns of agreement within the data were therefore used in the qualitative comparative analysis. Table 6 summarizes the six factors for each case.

TABLE 5.
SIXTEEN-FACTOR SUMMARY TABLE

	B*	C	D*	E	F	H*	J*	K	L	M	N	O	P*	Q*	T	U	Outcome
C1	0	0	0	1	0	1	0	1	0	1	1	0	0	0	1	0	F
A1	0	0	0	1	1	1	1	0	0	1	1	1	0	1	1	0	F
A3	1	1	0	1	1	1	1	0		0		1	0	1	0	0	F
A5	1	1	0	1	1	1	1	0		0		1	0	1	0	0	F
A7	1	1	0	1	1	1	1	0	1	0	1	1	0	1	0	1	F
U1	1	1	0	1	0	0	0	0	0	1	1	0	0	0	1	0	F
U2	1	1	0	1	0	0	0	0	0	1	1	0	0	1	0	0	F
U3	1	1	0	0	0	0	0	0	0	0	0	0	0	0	0	0	F
U4	1	1	0	1	0	0	1	0	0	0	0	0	0	1	0	0	F
U5	1	1	0	1	0	0	1	0	0	0	0	0	0	1	0	0	F
U6	1	1	0	0	0	0	1	0	0	0	0	0	0	1	0	1	F
U7	1	1	0	1	0	0	1	0	1	1	0	0	0	0	0	1	F
U8	1	1	0	0	0	0	1	0	1	1	0	0	0	0	0	1	F
C2	1	1	1	1	0	1	1	1	0	0	1	0	0	1	0	0	S
C3	1	1	1	1	0	1	1	1	1	0	0	0	1	1	0	1	S
C4	1	1	1	1	0	1	1	1	1	0	1	0	0	1	0	1	S
A2	1	0	0	1	1	1	1	0	0	1	1	1	1	1	1	0	S
A4	1	1	0	0	1	1	1	0	0	0		1	1	1	0	0	S
A6	1	1	0	1	1	1	1	0	1	0	0	1	1	1	0	1	S

A1–7 = Australian cases, C1–4 = Canadian cases, U1–8 = United States' cases.

F = NHI failure, S = NHI success. 0 = absent, 1 = present. *Selected factors.

B = federal health authority, C = federal health bureaucracy, D = lack of veto points, E = same-party majorities and executive, F = preferential voting or proportional representation, H = multiparty system, J = legislative legacy, K = hospital legacy, L = expenditure legacy, M = medical legacy, N = private insurance coverage, O = state corporatism, P = labor party power, Q = strong trade unions, T = political health industry, U = organized consumers.

All factors are measured so that "present" reflects the condition theorized to be conducive or "positive" for NHI.

TABLE 6.

SUMMARY TABLE OF THE SIX EMERGENT FACTORS BY OUTCOME TYPE

Cases	B Fed	D Veto	H Multi	J LL	P LP	Q Unions	Failure/ Success	Outcome Type
C1	0	0	1	0	0	0	F	(0)
A1	0	0	1	1	0	1	F	(0)
U1	1	0	0	0	0	0	F	(0)
U2	1	0	0	0	0	1	F	(0)
U3	1	0	0	0	0	0	F	0
U4	1	0	0	1	0	1	F	0
A3	1	0	1	1	0	1	F	P1
A5	1	0	1	1	0	1	F	P1
U5	1	0	0	1	0	1	F	P1
U6	1	0	0	1	0	1	F	P1
U7	1	0	0	1	0	0	F	P1
U8	1	0	0	1	0	0	F	P1
A7	1	0	1	1	0	1	F	P2
C2	1	1	1	1	0	1	S	P3
C3	1	1	1	1	1	1	S	P3
A2	1	0	1	1	1	1	S	P3
A4	1	0	1	1	1	1	S	P3
C4	1	1	1	1	0	1	S	PD
A6	1	0	1	1	1	1	S	PD

B/Fed = federal health authority, D/Veto = lack of veto points, H/Multi = multiparty system, J/LL = legislative legacy, P/LP = labor party power, Q/Unions = strong trade unions. P=public; PD=public and decommodifying; 0=neither. F = failure, S = success. A = Australia, C = Canada, U = United States.

APPENDIX D

*The Final Sixteen Factors and "Constants"**

Political Institutional Factors:

  †B. Federal authority or leverage with states/provinces in health care area‡

  C. Federal health bureaucracy

  †D. Veto points, other than federal constitutional authority in health area

  E. National executive and legislative majorities from the same party

  F. Preferential voting or proportional representation‡

  †H. A multiparty system

  †J. National or state/provincial hospital/medical programs‡

  K. Public management of hospitals for the public

  L. More public than private health expenditures

  M. Contract employment or public employment of M.D.s‡

  N. Less than half of citizens with private health insurance coverage

Power Resource Factors:

  O. Corporate state arrangements

  †P. Labor party in power, or in balance of power position in legislature‡

  †Q. Trade union strength 30 percent or greater

Interest-group Factors:

  T. No politically organized health industry‡

  U. Politically organized consumers

"Constants":

  Public ownership of hospitals (present / positive for all cases)

  Public subsidy of hospitals (present / positive for all cases)

  Other more decommodifying federal policies (absent / negative for all cases)

  No politically organized business lobbies (absent / negative for all cases)

  Politically active trade unions (present / positive for all cases)

  No politically organized medicine (absent / negative for all cases)

---

*To reduce confusion, all are measured so that present or positive (1) reflects the condition theorized as conducive for NHI; "absent" (0) therefore reflects a theoretically negative condition.

†the six emergent factors

‡variables formed by combining two related factors

APPENDIX E

A Short Introduction to Qualitative Comparative Analysis

Configurations (combinations of causal factors), rather than cases, are the basic unit of analysis in qualitative comparative analysis. The analysis examines combinations of relevant conditions from a data set, with outcomes, to determine which configurations produce the outcome of interest. Since a condition's absence may be theoretically important, negatives are included in configurations as well as positives.

For such an analysis, a summary of configurations rather than cases is needed. Boolean analysis therefore begins with the construction of a "truth table," a specialized form of summary table that systematically sets out all the possible configurations of a set of dichotomous (present or absent) variables and specifies an outcome for each configuration according to a data set. It is easiest to grasp the form and logic of a truth table in idealized form with a small number of factors. Using only three factors, an idealized truth table might look like table 7.

Each row of the truth table represents a single configuration. Any two cases with identical factor results exhibit the same configuration and are summarized in the same row. The total number of cases exhibiting each configuration is recorded in the right-hand column of its row. Truth tables help the analyst delineate and keep track of all possible configurations for a set of factors by setting the configurations out in a systematic fashion. They also facilitate the observation of patterns in the data.

The form of truth tables assures that if all causal conditions are included and accurately summarized in the table, each configuration will logically lead to a single outcome on the phenomenon of interest. In this representative truth table, as in this study, the outcomes are designated as success (S) or failure (F). In this table, it can be observed that the three configurations with successful outcomes (S) include, at a minimum, either factors B and C or factors A and C. In Boolean algebra, *and* is expressed as multiplication, while *or* is expressed as addition. The simplified Boolean "expression" for success for this table is therefore BC + AC = S, read as "B and C or A and C lead to S."

For many outcomes, expressions are lengthy, so simplifying methods have been devised to guide analysis. They utilize a specialized language, which is somewhat tedious but straightforward. As seen in the expression above, one letter is used for each factor; a capital letter signifies a 1 (or pos-

TABLE 7.
REPRESENTATIVE IDEALIZED TRUTH TABLE WITH THREE FACTORS

Factor A	Factor B	Factor C	Outcome	Number of Instances
0	0	0	F	3
0	0	1	F	3
0	1	0	F	1
0	1	1	S	1
1	0	0	F	7
1	0	1	S	3
1	1	0	F	1
1	1	1	S	3

0 = absent, 1 = present. F = failure, S = success. N = 22.

itive finding) for that condition for that configuration, and a small letter signifies a 0 (or negative finding). For example, the first row in the representative truth table exhibits the configuration F = abc, and the second row exhibits configuration F = abC. The right-hand column shows that both those configurations occurred in three cases or instances.

The Boolean expression for a specific outcome initially includes each full configuration leading to that outcome; that expression is then systematically reduced to its simplest logical form. The primary rule for reduction is that "if two Boolean expressions differ in only one causal condition yet produce the same outcome, then the causal condition that distinguishes the two expressions can be considered irrelevant and can be removed to create a simpler, combined expression" (Ragin 1987:93). For instance, if ABC + ABc = S, then the presence or absence of C is logically irrelevant to outcome S when both A and B are present, so AB = S. Once the initial expression is fully reduced, the result is an expression including only those factors that cannot be excluded as causal.

For the representative truth table, the initial expression would be S = aBC + AbC + ABC. Simplifying then proceeds step by step, by comparing each pair of configurations to see if reduction can take place. In this case, aBC and AbC are not reducible, because there are too many differences between them. However, since both aBC and ABC lead to S, then A must be irrelevant to S in the presence of B and C (i.e., if S = aBC + ABC, then S = BC). Similarly, since both AbC and ABC lead to S, then B must be irrelevant to S in the presence of A and C (i.e., if S = AbC + ABC, then

S = AC). The initial expression is therefore simplified to S = BC + AC. This reduced expression constitutes the result of the analysis, in that it summarizes the minimum specific combinations of factors from the data set that logically result in the outcome of interest.

In empirical studies, of course, truth tables are rarely as straightforward as is the idealized representative truth table provided. Some configurations may be found to result in both types of outcomes ("contradictory rows"), requiring some method to be devised for assigning specific outcomes to those configurations. In addition, empirical instances (cases) are rarely found for all configurations, and all configurations must be taken into account in the analysis in one way or another. While contradictory rows may indicate that important explanatory variables are missing, missing configurations constitute evidence that social phenomena occur in patterns, rather than randomly, and are in themselves potentially important data for analysis.

APPENDIX F

Tables used in the Qualitative Comparative Analysis

TABLE 8.
TRUTH TABLE FOR THE SIX EMERGENT FACTORS (CONDENSED)

B/Fed	D/Veto	H/Mult	J/LL	P/LP	Q/Unions	Outcome	#Instances
0	0	0	0	0	0	?	0
0	0	0	...			?	0
0	0	1	0	0	0	F	1 (C1)
0	0	1	...			?	0
0	0	1	1	0	1	F	1 (A1)
0	...					?	0
1	0	0	0	0	0	F	2 (U1&3)
1	0	0	0	0	1	F	1 (U2)
1	0	0	0	1	0	?	0
1	0	0	0	1	1	?	0
1	0	0	1	0	0	F	2 (U7&8)
1	0	0	1	0	1	F	3 (U4,5,6)
1	0	...				?	0
1	0	1	1	0	1	F	3(A3,5,7)
1	0	1	1	1	0	?	0
1	0	1	1	1	1	S	3 (A2,4,6)
1	1	...				?	0
1	1	1	1	0	1	S	2 (C2&4)
1	1	1	1	1	0	?	0
1	1	1	1	1	1	S	1 (C3)

B/Fed = federal power in health care area, D/Veto = lack of veto points, H/Mult = multi-party system, J/LL = legislative legacy, P/LP = labor party power, Q/Unions = strong trade unions. A = Australia, C = Canada, U = United States. 0 = absent, 1 = present. F = NHI failure, S = NHI success, ? = unknown.

TABLE 9.
TRUTH TABLE FOR THE TWO SUFFICIENT FACTORS

D/Veto	P/LP	Outcome	# Instances
0	0	F	13
0	1	S	3
1	0	S	2
1	1	S	1

D/Veto = lack of veto points, P/LP = labor party power.

0 = absent, 1 = present; F = NHI failure, S = NHI success.

TABLE 10.
TRUTH TABLE FOR THE FOUR NECESSARY CONDITIONS

B/Fed	H/Multi	J/LL	Q/Unions	Outcome	# Instances
0	0	0	0	?	0
0	0	0	1	?	0
0	0	1	0	?	0
0	0	1	1	?	0
0	1	0	0	F	1
0	1	0	1	?	0
0	1	1	0	?	0
0	1	1	1	F	1
1	0	0	0	F	2
1	0	0	1	F	1
1	0	1	0	F	2
1	0	1	1	F	3
1	1	0	0	?	0
1	1	0	1	?	0
1	1	1	0	?	0
1	1	1	1	S	9 (6S, 3F)

B/Fed = federal power in health care area, H/Multi = multiparty system, J/LL = legislative legacy, Q/Unions = strong trade unions.

0 = absent, 1 = present. F = NHI failure, S = NHI success, ? = unknown.

TABLE 11. SUMMARY TABLE BY NATION

	B Fed	D Veto	H Multi	J LL	P LP	Q Unions	Failure/ Success	Outcome (Type)
C1	0	0	1	0	0	0	F	(0)
C2	1	1	1	1	0	1	S	P3
C3	1	1	1	1	1	1	S	P3
C4	1	1	1	1	0	1	S	PD
A1	0	0	1	1	0	1	F	(0)
A2	1	0	1	1	1	1	S	P3
A3	1	0	1	1	0	1	F	P1
A4	1	0	1	1	1	1	S	P3
A5	1	0	1	1	0	1	F	P1
A6	1	0	1	1	1	1	S	PD
A7	1	0	1	1	0	1	F	P2
U1	1	0	0	0	0	0	F	(0)
U2	1	0	0	0	0	1	F	(0)
U3	1	0	0	0	0	0	F	0
U4	1	0	0	1	0	1	F	0
U5	1	0	0	1	0	1	F	P1
U6	1	0	0	1	0	1	F	P1
U7	1	0	0	1	0	0	F	P1
U8	1	0	0	1	0	0	F	P1

B/Fed = federal power in health care area, D/Veto = lack of veto points, H/Multi = multi-party system, J/LL = legislative legacy, P/LP = labor party power, Q/Unions = strong trade unions. P= public; PD = public and decommodifying; 0 = neither.

A = Australia, C = Canada, U = United States. 0 = absent, 1 = present. F = failure, S = success.

Notes

INTRODUCTION

1. None of the nations in this study have instituted, or come close to instituting, programs in which health services are taken over and run by the state. For this reason, and to simplify the discussion, *national health insurance* (NHI) is used to refer to both national health service and insurance programs in these nations.

2. The power resources theoretical tradition has often been referred to in the U.S. welfare state literature as "social democratic theory" (see Pampel and Williamson 1988; Esping-Andersen and van Kersbergen 1992; Huber et al. 1993). However, this usage rather misleadingly conflates an explanatory theory with the political goal of some (but not all) working-class activists. Concurrently with this usage, the more specifically delineated power resources theory has come to represent this theoretical tradition in the theoretical and international welfare state literature (see Korpi 1985; O'Connor and Olsen 1998; Bradley et al. 2003). In this book, *power resources theory* will be used for the theoretical tradition, and *social democratic* for the political goal and the actors/parties that promote it.

3. Social democratic, labor, and socialist parties can, of course, be deliberately mislabeled or taken over by members with other goals, so party names should never be assumed to accurately represent political agendas.

4. The idea of concessions is generally associated with structural Marxism, which presumes that policies adopted under such circumstances will actually strengthen capitalism and do little for the working class. However, where that presumption is absent, so that the resulting policies may be evaluated on their empirical effects, this idea is not necessarily incompatible with power resources theory. In particular, the imbalance in power resources in a state where the working class is very weak may produce the dynamics described by mass turmoil theory. This possibility appears supported by the primary focus of such theorists on the United States (Olsen 2002:124–25). In such states, because it raises the costs of both business and politics as usual, unorganized agitation may serve as a type of power resource.

5. Commodification is the act of turning something into a saleable commodity, and decommodification is the act of turning a saleable commodity into

something else. In health care, decommodification means separating access to care from the ability to pay for it.

6. This approach has been challenged recently by welfare state theorists who emphasize the family as a private source of social provision and suggest the importance of gender and race as well as class in categorizing welfare states (O'Connor et al. 1999). However, these ideas have not yet been incorporated into a coherent set of analytical categories.

CHAPTER 3. AUSTRALIA

1. The Australian Medical Association was called the "British Medical Association" in Australia until 1962. In the interests of clarity, however, the term *Australian Medical Association* (AMA) is used throughout the narrative.

CHAPTER 5. A SECOND, SYSTEMATIC APPROACH

1. A good deal of debate has occurred over the specific nature of classes, their number, and what groups belong to each class. For the purposes of this book, the term *dominant class* will be used to signify the upper class and those members of the corporate community who share the upper class's power, privilege, and interest in preserving structural inequities at a given point in time (Domhoff 2002). The terms *working class* and *subordinate class* will be used to signify those dependent upon either employment or welfare state policies for their access to health care and other goods at a given point in time. While there appears to be some overlap in the two categories, the extent of this overlap and the precise class position of citizens caught in it are not critical factors for this study. A recent discussion of class categorization issues can be found in the *American Journal of Sociology*, 105, no. 6, 2000, pp. 1523–82.

2. These criteria and discussion are based upon Esping-Andersen's three welfare state characteristics of stratification, public/private mix, and commodification. In the nations examined in this work, the basis for stratification in welfare state policies is commodification; stratification would therefore duplicate commodification as a criteria. For that reason, only two of the three criteria are used in this study.

3. The finding of empirical outcomes for only 10 of the 64 possible configurations supports the presumption that there are only a few ways in which causal factors produce NHI success or failure in these nations. It also establishes boundaries to the results of this study, which cannot be considered definitive for nations that exhibit different configurations and outcomes.

4. For instance, when the criteria (S = BDQ + BPQ) is used to assign outcomes to not-found configurations, the result is the reduced expression (S = BDQ + BPQ), and when the assignment criteria (S = BP + BD) is used, the result is (S = BP + BD). This is a logical result when there are more assigned than empirical outcomes in the data analyzed. (See appendices D and E for a list of the factors assigned to these letters and an introduction to this language.)

5. Since causation occurs in patterns, it is highly unlikely that all those configurations specifically missing from an empirical study could occur. Furthermore, the proportion of failed to successful attempts to pass NHI found in this study casts considerable doubt on the likelihood that the missing configurations could produce more NHI success than failure.

6. Logically, such a dynamic could take two forms, exhibiting either no shared factors (S = ABC + DEF), or both shared and unshared factors (S = ABD + ABE). The first of these involves no overlap in the factors on each path; the second involves one or more factors necessary on all paths to the outcome of interest, plus at least two factors that distinguish the paths from each other. The second of these forms was found in this study.

CHAPTER 6. CONCLUSIONS

1. However, the relation between the four necessary conditions and the two sufficient conditions remains unknown and could logically be additive rather than interactive in nature.

APPENDICES

1. One case is noted to have had policy outcomes different than the other cases in the same table cell or those that would be logically expected in that cell. Case A4 is noted to have had fewer decommodifying effects than its provisions warranted. The fact that Labor's Medibank policy was in effect only a few months in Australia before it was significantly changed by the incoming Liberal government appears to have prevented Medibank from removing market-based divisions in the quality of care available to citizens, as the nearly identical Medicare program did later.

Bibliography

Aaron, Henry J. (1991). *Serious and Unstable Condition: Financing America's Health Care.* Washington, D.C.: Brookings Institute.

Abbott, Maude E. (1931). *History of Medicine in the Province of Quebec.* Montreal: McGill University.

Agar, Herbert (1966). *The Price of Union: The Influence of the American Temper on the Course of History.* Boston: Houghton Mifflin.

AHA News (2001). "Switch from Medicaid to SCHIP Often Leaves Children Uncovered." 37, 24: 8.

Aitkin, Don and Brian Jinks (1982). *Australian Political Institutions.* Carlton, Victoria: Pitman.

Alber, Jens, Gosta Esping-Andersen, and Lee Rainwater (1987). In *Comparative Policy Research: Learning From Experience*, Meinolf Dierkes, Hans N. Weiler, and Ariane Berthoin Antal, eds., New York: St. Martin's, 1987, pp. 458–69.

Alford, Robert R. (1973). *Party and Society: The Anglo-American Democracies.* Westport, Conn.: Greenwood.

——— (1975). *Health Care Politics: Ideological and Interest Group Barriers to Reform.* Chicago: University of Chicago Press.

Allen, Donna (1971). "Inadequate Media and the Failure of the National Health Insurance Proposal in the Late 1940s." Ph.D. thesis. Howard University, Washington, D.C.

Amenta, Edwin and Jane D. Poulsen (1994). "Where to Begin: A Survey of Five Approaches to Selecting Independent Variables for Qualitative Comparative Analysis." *Sociological Methods & Research*, 23, 1, pp. 22–53.

American Academy of Pediatrics, Department of Chapter and State Affairs (2000). "Summary of Title XXI Programs in States" (cited on July 30, 2002). Available online at http://www.aap.org/advocacy/txxisummary.pdf.

Anderson, Odin W. (1968). *The Uneasy Equilibrium: Private and Public Financing of Health Services in the United States, 1875–1965.* New Haven, Conn.: College & University Press.

——— (1990). *Health Services as a Growth Enterprise in the United States Since 1875.* Ann Arbor: Health Administration.

Andrews, Margaret W. (1981). "Medical Attendence in Vancouver, 1886–1920." In *Medicine in Canadian Society: Historical Perspectives*, S.E.D. Shortt, ed., Montreal: McGill-Queen's University Press, pp. 417–45.

Australian Labor Party (1980). "The Relationship between the Australian Labor Party and the Trade Unions." Discussion Paper.

Badgley, Robin F. and Samuel Wolfe (1967). *Doctors' Strike: Medical Care and Conflict in Saskatchewan*. New York: Atherton.

———— (1992). "Equity and Health Care." In *Canadian Health Care and the State: A Century of Evolution*, C. David Naylor, ed., Montreal: McGill-Queen's University Press, pp. 193–238.

Baldwin, Peter (1989). "The Scandinavian Origins of the Social Interpretation of the Welfare State." *Comparative Studies in Society and History*, 31, 1, 3–24.

Banting, Keith (1997). "The Social Policy Divide: The Welfare State in Canada and the United States." In *Degrees of Freedom: Canada and the United States in a Changing World*, Keith Banting, George Hoberg, and Richard Simeon, eds., Montreal & Kingston: McGill-Queen's University Press, pp. 267–309.

Behan, Pamela (1998). "Ideology and Health Policy: Cultural Roots of the Managed Care Debate." Paper presented at the annual meetings of the American Sociological Association, San Francisco, August 23.

———— (2000). "Political Institutions and the Democratic Class Struggle: The Politics of National Health Insurance in the United States, Canada and Australia." Ph.D. dissertation, University of Colorado, Boulder.

Bell, David V. J. (1992). *The Roots of Disunity: A Study of Canadian Political Culture*. Toronto: Oxford University Press.

Bergthold, Linda A. (1995). "American Business and Health Care Reform: 'Do We Have to Move So Fast?'" Paper presented at the annual meetings of the American Sociological Association, Washington, D.C., August 21.

Bjelke-Petersen, Joh (1983). "Australian Federalism: A Queensland View." In *Australian Federalism: Future Tense*, Allan Patience and Jeffrey Scott, eds., Melbourne: Oxford University Press, pp. 63–74.

Blake, Charles H. and Jessica R. Adolino (2001). "The Enactment of National Health Insurance: A Boolean Analysis of Twenty Advanced Industrial Countries." *Journal of Health Politics, Policy and Law*, 26, 4, 679–708.

Blankenau, Joe (2001). "The Fate of National Health Insurance in Canada and the United States: A Multiple Streams Explanation." *Policy Studies Journal*, 29, 1, 38–55.

Blendon, Robert J. (1989). "Three Systems: A Comparative Survey." *Health Management Quarterly*, 11, 1, 2–10.

Boase, Joan (1996). "Institutions, Institutionalized Networks and Policy Choices: Health Policy in the U.S and Canada." *Government and Opposition*, 9, 3, 287–310.

Bothwell, Robert S. (1977). "The Health of the Common People." In *Mackenzie King: Widening the Debate*, John English and J. O. Stubbs, eds., Toronto: Macmillan of Canada, pp. 191–220.

Bradley, David, Evelyne Huber, Stephanie Moller, Francois Nielsen, and John D. Stephens (2003). "Distribution and Redistribution in Postindustrial Democracies." *World Politics*, 55, 2, 193–228.

Brown, Nona (1956). "Federal Health Program Puts Accent on Research: Private Agencies Expand Insurance but Many Persons Are Still Not Covered." From *The New York Times*, Jan. 29, 4: 10.

Business Week (1970). "$60–Billion Crisis in Health Care." January 17, pp. 50–64.

Butlin, N. G., A. Barnard, and J. J. Pincus (1982). *Government and Capitalism: Public and Private Choice in Twentieth Century Australia*. Sydney: Allen & Unwin.

Byck, Gayle R. (2000). "A Comparison of the Socioeconomic and Health Status Characteristics of Uninsured, State Children's Health Insurance Program-Eligible Children in the United States with Those of Other Groups of Insured Children: Implications for Policy." *Pediatrics*, 106, 1:14–21.

Caiden, Gerald E. (1966). "The A.C.P.T.A.: A Study of White Collar Public Service Unionism in the Commonwealth of Australia 1885–1922." Occasional Papers No. 2, Department of Political Science, Research School of Social Sciences, Australian National University, Canberra.

Canada. Department of National Health and Welfare. Research and Statistics Division (1955). *Selected Public Hospital and Medical Care Plans in Canada*. Social Security Series, Memorandum No. 15. Ottawa: Department of National Health and Welfare.

——— (1957). *Voluntary Hospital and Medical Insurance in Canada, 1955: Summary Data*. Health Care Series No. 6. Ottawa: Department of National Health and Welfare.

Canada. Royal Commission on Health Services (1964). Report (Hall Report), vol. 1. Ottawa: Queen's Printer.

Chaison, Gary N. and Joseph B. Rose (1991). "The Macrodeterminants of Union Growth and Decline." In *The State of the Unions*, George Strauss, Daniel G. Gallagher, and Jack Fiorito, eds., Madison, Wisconsin: Industrial Relations Research Association, pp. 3–45.

Charles, Cathy and Robin F. Badgley (1997). "National Health Insurance: Evolution and Unresolved Policy Issues." Unpublished paper; to be published in *Health Care Reform: International Perspectives*, F. D. Powell and A. F. Wesson, eds., Sage.

Chesterman, Esther (1986). "Discussion." In *Economics and Health 1985: Proceedings of the Seventh Australian Conference of Health Economists*, James R. G. Butler and Darrel P. Doessel, eds., Kensington: School of Health Administration, University of New South Wales, pp. 79–80.

Chi, N. H. and G. C. Perlin (1979). "The New Democratic Party: A Party in Transition." From *Party Politics in Canada*, Hugh G. Thorburn, ed., Scarborough, Ont.: Prentice-Hall of Canada, 1979, pp. 177–87.

Christian, William and Colin Campbell (1983). *Political Parties and Ideologies in Canada: Liberals, Conservatives, Socialists, Nationalists*. Toronto: McGraw-Hill Ryerson.

Clarke, Cal and Rene McEldowney (2000). "The Performance of National Health Care Systems: A 'Good News, Bad News' Finding for Reform Possibilities." *Policy Studies Review*, 17, 4, pp. 133–48.

Crichton, Anne (1990). *Slowly Taking Control? Australian Governments and Health Care Provision, 1788–1988*. Sydney: Allen & Unwin.

Dahl, Robert A. (1956). *A Preface to Democratic Theory*. Chicago: University of Chicago Press.

——— (1986). *Democracy, Liberty and Equality*. Oslo: Norwegian University Press.

Deeble, J. S. (1982). "Financing Health Care in a Static Economy." *Social Science and Medicine*, 16: 713–24.

Delaney, John Thomas and Marick F. Masters (1991). "Unions and Political Action." In *The State of the Unions*, George Strauss, Daniel G. Gallagher, and Jack Fiorito, eds., Madison, Wisconsin: Industrial Relations Research Association, pp. 313–45.

Dickey, Brian (1980). *No Charity There: A Short History of Social Welfare in Australia*. Melbourne: Nelson Australia.

Domhoff, G. William (1995). "Who Killed Health Care Reform in Congress, Small Business or Rich Conservatives, and Why Did They Do It?" Paper presented at the annual meetings of the American Sociological Association in Washington, D.C., August 21.

——— (2002). *Who Rules America?* St. Louis: McGraw Hill.

Drass, Kriss A. (1992). *Qualitative Comparative Analysis 3.0*. Evanston, Illinois: Center for Urban Affairs and Policy Research, Northwestern University.

Durkheim, Emile (1983). *Professional Ethics and Civic Morals*. Cornelia Brookfield, translator. Westport, Conn.: Greenwood.

Elola, Javier, Antonio Daponte, and Vicente Navarro (1995). "Health Indicators and the Organization of Health Care Systems in Western Europe." *American Journal of Public Health*, 85: 1397–1401.

Esman, Milton J. (1984). "Federalism and Modernization: Canada and the United States." *Publius: The Journal of Federalism*, 14: 21–38.

Esping-Andersen, Gøsta (1985). *Politics against Markets: The Social Democratic Road to Power*. Princeton: Princeton University Press.

——— (1990). *The Three Worlds of Welfare Capitalism*. Princeton, New Jersey: Princeton University Press.

Esping-Andersen, Gøsta and Kees van Kersbergen (1992). "Contemporary Research on Social Democracy." *Annual Review of Sociology*, 18:187–208.

Evans, Robert G. (1988). "'We'll Take Care of It for You:' Health Care in the Canadian Community." *Daedalus*, 117, 4, 155–89.

Fain, Tyrus G., Katherine C. Plant, and Ross Milloy, eds. (1977). *National Health Insurance*. New York: Bowker.

Fein, Rashi (1986). *Medical Care, Medical Costs: The Search for a Health Insurance Policy*. Cambridge: Harvard University Press.

Financing and Analysis Branch, Commonwealth Department of Health and Aging (2000). "The Australian Health Care System: An Outline—September 2000" (cited on July 11, 2002). Available online at http://www.health.gov.au/haf/ozhealth/ozhcsyspart3.htm.

Foenander, Orwell de R. (1937). *Towards Industrial Peace in Australia: A Series of Essays in the History of the Commonwealth Court of Conciliation and Arbitration.* Melbourne: Melbourne University Press.

Ford, Gerald R. (1975). "Address to the Nation." *Weekly Compilation of Presidential Documents*, Washington, D.C.: Office of the Federal Register, Jan. 13.

Forsey, Eugene (1985). "The History of the Canadian Labour Movement." In *Lectures in Canadian Labour and Working-Class History*, W. J. C. Cherwinski and G. S. Kealey, eds., St. John's, Newfoundland: Committee on Labour History and New Hogtown Press, 7–22.

Fortune (1970). "It's Time to Operate." January, p. 79.

Fox, Daniel M. (1986). *Health Policies, Health Politics: The British and American Experience, 1911–1965.* Princeton, New Jersey: Princeton University Press.

Frenkel, Stephen J. (1988). "Australian Employers in the Shadow of the Labor Accords." *Industrial Relations*, 27, 2 (Spring), pp. 166–79.

Fry, Eric, ed. (1986). *Common Cause: Essays in Australia and New Zealand Labour History.* Wellington: Allen & Unwin/Port Nicholson.

Fuchs, Victor (1986). *The Health Economy.* Cambridge: Harvard University Press.

Ganguly, Rajat (1997). "The Move towards Disintegration: Explaining Ethnosecessionist Mobilization in South Asia." *Nationalism and Ethnic Politics*, 3, 2 (Summer), 101–30.

Gardner, Heather, ed. (1995). *The Politics of Health: The Australian Experience.* Melbourne: Churchill Livingstone.

Gay, Peter (1968). "The Enlightenment." In *The Comparative Approach to American History*, C. Vann Woodward, ed., New York: Basic Books, pp. 34–46.

Gibb, George D. (1855). *The Journal of Public Health* (UK), 1, 2. Reprinted in *Canadian Journal of Public Health*, 85, 3, p. 149.

Gibbins, Roger (1982). *Regionalism: Territorial Politics in Canada and the United States.* Toronto: Butterworths.

Gillespie, James A. (1991). *The Price of Health: Australian Governments and Medical Politics 1910–60.* Cambridge: Cambridge University Press.

Ginzberg, Eli (1977). *The Limits of Health Reform: The Search for Realism.* New York: Basic Books.

Godfrey, Charles M. (1979). *Medicine for Ontario: A History.* Belleville, Ontario: Mika.

Gottschalk, Marie (2000). *The Shadow Welfare State: Labor, Business, and the Politics of Health Care in the United States.* Ithaca: IRL.

Grant, Vicki C. (1992). "An Analysis of the Reasons National Health Insurance Failed to Become Policy in the United States." Ph.D. thesis. Florence Heller Graduate School for Advanced Studies in Social Welfare, Brandeis University, Waltham, Massachusetts.

Gray, Gwendolyn (1984). "The Termination of Medibank." *Politics*, 19, 2, 1–17.

——— (1987). "Privatisation: An Attempt that Failed." *Politics*, 22, 2, 15–28.

——— (1990). "Health Policy." In *Hawke and Australian Public Policy: Consensus and Restructuring*, Christine Jennett and Randal G. Stewart, eds., Melbourne: MacMillan, pp. 223–44.

——— (1991). *Federalism and Health Policy: The Development of Health Systems in Canada and Australia.* Toronto: University of Toronto Press.

Green, David G. and Lawrence G. Cromwell (1984). *Mutual Aid or Welfare State: Australia's Friendly Societies.* Sydney: Allen & Unwin.

Hage, Jerald and J. Rogers Hollingsworth (1995). "Clinton Health Care Reform and the Diminishment of the Active State." Paper presented at the annual meetings of the American Sociological Association in Washington, D.C., August 21.

Hanneman, Robert and J. Rogers Hollingsworth (1992). "Refocusing the Debate on the Role of the State in Capitalist Societies." In *State Theory and State History*, Rolf Torstendahl, ed., London: Sage, 38–61.

Hartz, Louis (1964). *The Founding of New Societies: Studies in the History of the United States, Latin America, South Africa, Canada, and Australia.* New York: Harcourt, Brace & World.

Heagerty, John J. (1928). *Four Centuries of Medical History in Canada.* 2 volumes. Toronto: MacMillan Canada.

Heclo, Hugh (1974). *Modern Social Politics in Britain and Sweden.* New Haven, Conn.: Yale University Press.

Hertzberg, Hedrick (1991). "Making Tracks Toward '92." *Los Angeles Times*, November 10, p. M1.

Hicks, Alexander (1994). "Qualitative Comparative Analysis and Analytical Induction: The Case of the Emergence of the Social Security State." *Sociological Methods and Research*, 23, 1, 86–113.

Hicks, Alexander and Joya Misra (1993). "Two Perspectives on the Welfare State: Political Resources and the Growth of Welfare in Affluent Capitalist Democracies, 1960–1982." *American Journal of Sociology*, 99: 668–710.

Hicks, Alexander, Joya Misra, and Tang Nah Ng (1995). "The Programmatic Emergence of the Social Security State." *American Sociological Review*, 60: 329–49.

Hirshfield, Daniel S. (1970). *The Lost Reform: The Campaign for Compulsory Health Insurance in the United States from 1932 to 1943.* Cambridge, Mass.: Harvard University Press.

Hoffman, Beatrix (2001). *The Wages of Sickness: The Politics of Health Insurance in Progressive America.* Chapel Hill: University of North Carolina Press.

Horowitz, Gad (1966). "Conservatism, Liberalism, and Socialism in Canada: An Interpretation." *The Canadian Journal of Economics and Political Science*, 32, 2, pp. 143–71.

——— (1968). *Canadian Labour in Politics.* Toronto: University of Toronto Press.

Houseman, Gerald Laverne (1971). "Trade Unions and the Australian Labor Party: A Study of the Political Consequences of Affiliation." Ph.D. Dissertation, Department of Political Science, University of Illinois, Urbana-Champaign.

Howell, Colin D. (1992). "Medical Science and Social Criticism: Alexander Peter Reid and the Ideological Origins of the Welfare State in Canada." In *Canadian Health Care and the State: A Century of Evolution*, C. David Naylor, ed., Montreal: McGill-Queen's University Press, pp. 16–37.

Huber, Evelyne, Charles Ragin and John D. Stephens (1993). "Social Democracy, Christian Democracy, Constitutional Structure and the Welfare State." *American Journal of Sociology*, 99, 3, 711–49.

Hunter, Thelma (1980). "Pressure Groups and the Australian Political Process: The Case of the Australian Medical Association." *The Journal of Commonwealth and Comparative Politics*, 18, 2, pp. 190–206.

Hurley, Jeremiah and Steven Morgan (2004). "U.S. Medicare Reform: Why Drug Companies and Private Insurers Are Smiling." *Canadian Medical Association Journal*, 170, 4 (February 17), 461–62.

Immergut, Ellen M. (1990). "Institutions, Veto Points, and Policy Results: A Comparative Analysis of Health Care." *Journal of Public Policy*, 10: 391–416.

——— (1992a). "The Rules of the Game: The Logic of Health Policy-making in France, Switzerland, and Sweden." In *Structuring Politics: Historical Institutionalism in Comparative Analysis*, Sven Steinmo, Kathleen Thelen and Frank Longstreth, eds., New York: Cambridge University Press, 1992, pp. 57–89.

——— (1992b). *Health Politics: Interests and Institutions in Western Europe*. New York: Cambridge University Press.

Jaensch, Dean (1994). *Power Politics: Australia's Party System*. St. Leonards, New South Wales: Allen & Unwin.

Jennett, Christine and Randal G. Stewart (1990). *Hawke and Australian Public Policy: Consensus and Restructuring*. Melbourne: Macmillan of Australia.

Jensen, Merrill (1968). "The Colonial Phase." In *The Comparative Approach to American History*, C. Vann Woodward, ed., New York: Basic Books, 1968, 18–33.

Jones, M. A. (1983). *The Australian Welfare State: Growth, Crisis and Change*. Sydney: Allen & Unwin.

Kemper, Vicki (2004). "Few Seniors Understand Changes to Medicare." *Los Angeles Times*; reprinted in *The Houston Chronicle*, February 27.

Kennedy, Richard, ed. (1982). *Australian Welfare History: Critical Essays*. Melbourne: Macmillan of Australia.

Korpi, Walter (1983). *The Democratic Class Struggle*. London: Routledge & Kegan Paul.

——— (1985). "Power Resources Approach vs. Action and Conflict: On Causal and Intentional Explanations in the Study of Power." *Sociological Theory*, 3, 2, 31–35. Reprinted in *Power Resources Theory and the Welfare State: A Critical Approach*, Julia S. O'Connor and Gregg M. Olsen, eds., Toronto: University of Toronto Press, 1998, pp. 37–69.

——— (1998). "The Iceberg of Power below the Surface: A Preface to Power Resources Theory." In *Power Resources Theory and the Welfare State: A Critical Approach*, Julia S. O'Connor and Gregg M. Olsen, eds., Toronto: University of Toronto Press, pp. vii–xiv.

Kosterlitz, Julie (1992). "A Sick System." *National Journal*. February 15.

Kramer, Michael (1991). "The Voters' Latest Ailment: Health Care." *Time*, November 11, p. 51.

Kunitz, Stephen J. (1992). "Socialism and Social Insurance in the United States and Canada." In *Canadian Health Care and the State: A Century of Evolution*, C. David Naylor, ed., Montreal: McGill-Queen's University Press, pp. 104–24.

Laham, Nicholas (1992). "The Elusive Reform: The Politics of National Health Insurance 1915–1991." Ph.D. dissertation. Claremont Graduate School, Claremont, California.

——— (1993). *Why the United States Lacks a National Health Insurance Program*. Westport, Conn.: Greenwood.

——— (1996). *A Lost Cause: Bill Clinton's Campaign for National Health Insurance*. Westport, Conn.: Praeger.

Larkin, John (1989). "The New South Wales Doctors' Dispute 1984–85: An Interpretation." *Politics*, 24, 2, November, pp. 67–78.

Light, Donald (2002). Public statement at a Section on Medical Sociology paper session entitled "Toward Universal Access to Quality Health Care," American Sociological Association meetings, Chicago, Illinois, August 17.

Lipset, Seymour Martin (1971 [1950]). *Agrarian Socialism: The Cooperative Commonwealth Federation in Saskatchewan*. Berkeley: University of California Press.

——— (1967). *The First New Nation: The United States in Historical and Comparative Perspective*. Garden City, New York: Anchor Books.

——— (1989). *Continental Divide: The Values and Institutions of the United States and Canada*. Toronto: Howe Institute.

Logan, H. A. (1948). *Trade Unions in Canada: Their Development and Functioning*. Toronto: MacMillan of Canada.

Macarthy, P. G. (1970). "The Living Wage in Australia: The Role of Government." *Labour History*, 18, May, pp. 3–18.

Machado, Arthur Franco (1985). "National Health Insurance: Revelations in Congressional Testimony." Ph.D. dissertation. University of Nebraska, Lincoln.

Mackay, Relief (1981). "Poor Relief and Medicine in Nova Scotia, 1749–83." In *Medicine in Canadian Society: Historical Perspectives*, S. E. D. Shortt, ed., Montreal: McGill-Queen's University Press, pp. 75–92.

MacPherson, Ian (1979). *The Co-Operative Movement on the Prairies, 1900–55*. Canada Historical Association Booklets, No. 33. Ottawa: Love.

Maioni, Antonia (1998). *Parting at the Crossroads: The Emergence of Health Insurance in the United States and Canada*. Princeton: Princeton University Press.

Markey, Ray (1982). "The A.L.P. and the Emergence of a National Social Policy, 1880–1910." In *Australian Welfare History: Critical Essays*, Richard Kennedy, ed., Melbourne: Macmillan of Australia.

Marmor, Theodore R. and Jon B. Christianson (1982). *Health Care Policy: A Political Economy Approach*. Beverly Hills: Sage.

Marsh, Ian (1995). *Beyond the Two Party System: Political Representation, Economic Competitiveness and Australian Politics*. Cambridge: Cambridge University Press.

Marshall, T. H. (1964). *Class, Citizenship, and Social Development: Essays by T. H. Marshall.* Westport, Conn.: Greenwood.

Martin, E. W. (1972). *Comparative Development in Social Welfare.* London: Allen & Unwin.

Martin, Paul (1977). "King: the View from the Backbench and the Cabinet Table." In *Mackenzie King: Widening the Debate*, John English and J. O. Stubbs, eds., Toronto: Macmillan of Canada, pp. 30–39.

Martin, R. M. (1966–7). "Australian Trade Unions and Political Action." *Parliamentary Affairs*, 20, 1 (Winter), pp. 35–48.

Mathis, Paul C. (1970). "A Comparison of Canadian and U.S. Labor Movements." *Michigan Academician*, 3, 2 (Fall), pp. 33–43.

McConnell, Grant (1967). *Private Power and American Democracy.* New York: Knopf.

McInnis, Edgar (1959). *Canada: A Political and Social History.* New York: Holt, Rinehart & Winston.

McKay, B. V. (1986). "A Participant's Account of the New South Wales Doctor's Dispute." *Community Health Studies*, 10, 2, pp. 220–31.

Mental Health Weekly (2002). "States Cutting Back on CHIP." 12, 10:7.

Mills, John Stuart ([1843] 1967). *A System of Logic: Ratiocinative and Inductive.* Toronto: University of Toronto Press.

Mintz, Beth (1998). "The Failure of Health-Care Reform: The Role of Big Business in Policy Formation." In *Social Policy and the Conservative Agenda*, Clarence Y. H. Lo and Michael Schwartz, eds., Oxford: Blackwell, pp. 210–24.

Mishra, Ramesh (1990). *The Welfare State in Capitalist Society: Policies of Retrenchment and Maintenance in Europe, North America and Australia.* Toronto: University of Toronto Press.

Mitchell, Ross (1954). *Medicine in Manitoba: The Story of Its Beginnings.* Winnipeg: Stovel-Advocate.

Moran, Michael (2000). "Understanding the Welfare State: The Case of Health Care." *British Journal of Politics and International Relations*, 2, 2, pp. 135–60.

Morone, James A. (1990). *The Democratic Wish: Popular Participation and the Limits of American Government.* Basic Books.

——— (1993). "The Bureaucracy Empowered." In *The Politics of Health Care Reform: Lessons from the Past, Prospects for the Future*, James A. Morone and Gary S. Belkin, eds., Durham: Duke University Press, 1994, pp. 148–64.

Morris, Jonas (1985). *Searching for a Cure: National Health Policy Considered.* Washington, D.C.: Berkeley Morgan.

Mulgan, Richard (1994). *Politics in New Zealand.* Auckland: Auckland University Press.

Navarro, Vicente (1989). "Why Some Countries Have National Health Insurance, Others Have National Health Services, and the United States Has Neither." *Social Science and Medicine*, 28: 887–98.

——— (1992). *Why the United States Does Not Have a National Health Program.* Amityville, N.Y.: Baywood.

Naylor, C. David, ed. (1992). *Canadian Health Care and the State: A Century of Evolution*. Montreal: McGill-Queen's University Press.

Neatby, Hilda (1981). "The Medical Profession in the North-West Territories." In *Medicine in Canadian Society: Historical Perspectives*, S. E. D. Shortt, ed., Montreal: McGill-Queen's University Press, pp. 165–88.

New Democratic Party (1976). *New Democratic Policies 1961–1976*. Ottawa: Mutual.

The New York Times (1958). "Gaps in Health Insurance." September 15, p. 20.

O'Connor, Julia S. and Greg M. Olsen, eds. (1998). *Power Resources Theory and the Welfare State: A Critical Approach*. Toronto: University of Toronto Press.

O'Connor, Julia S., Ann Shola Orloff, and Sheila Shaver (1999). *States, Markets, Families: Gender, Liberalism, and Social Policy in Australia, Canada, Great Britain, and the United States*. Cambridge: Cambridge University Press.

Offe, C. (1984). *Contradictions of the Welfare State*. Cambridge, Mass.: MIT Press.

Olsen, Gregg M. (1992). *The Struggle for Economic Democracy in Sweden*. Avebury: Aldershot.

——— (1994). "Locating the Canadian Welfare State: Family Policy and Health Care in Canada, Sweden and the United States." *Canadian Journal of Sociology*, 19, 1, 1–20.

——— (2002). *The Politics of the Welfare State: Canada, Sweden and the United States*. Toronto: Oxford University Press.

Olsen, Gregg M. and Julia S. O'Connor (1998). "Understanding the Welfare State: Power Resources Theory and Its Critics." In *Power Resources Theory and the Welfare State: A Critical Approach*, Julia S. O'Connor and Gregg M. Olsen, eds., Toronto: University of Toronto Press, pp. 3–33.

Orloff, Ann Shola (1993). *The Politics of Pensions: A Comparative Analysis of Britain, Canada, and the United States, 1880–1940*. Madison: University of Wisconsin Press.

Ostry, Aleck (1994). "Saskatchewan's Unique Rural Public Health Tradition." *Canadian Journal of Public Health*, 85, 4, p. 222.

Palmer, George R. and Stephanie D. Short (1989). *Health Care and Public Policy: An Australian Analysis*. Melbourne: Macmillan of Australia.

Pampel, Fred C. (1994). "Population Aging, Class Context, and Age Inequality in Public Spending." *American Journal of Sociology*, 100: 153–95.

Pampel, Fred C. and John B. Williamson (1988). "Welfare Spending in Advanced Industrial Democracies." *American Journal of Sociology*, 93, 6, 1424–56.

Parenti, Michael (1986). *Inventing Reality: The Politics of the Mass Media*. New York: St. Martin's.

Pear, Robert (2003). "Watershed Medicare Bill Signed." *The New York Times*; reprinted in *The Houston Chronicle*, December 9, 1A.

——— (2004). "AARP Seeks Changes in New Medicare Law: Wants to Make Drugs More Affordable." *The New York Times*; reprinted in *The Houston Chronicle*, January 17, 21A.

Pensabene, Tony S. (1986). "Implications of the New South Wales Doctors' Dispute." In *Economics and Health 1985: Proceedings of the Seventh Australian Conference of Health Economists*, James R. G. Butler and Darrel P. Doessel, eds., Kensington: School of Health Administration, University of New South Wales, pp. 67–78.

Peterson, Mark A. (1993). "Congress in the 1990's: From Iron Triangles to Policy Networks." In *The Politics of Health Care Reform: Lessons from the Past, Prospects for the Future*, James A. Morone and Gary S. Belkin, eds., Durham: Duke University Press, 1994, pp. 103–47.

Pickersgill, J. W. (1977). "Mackenzie King's Political Attitudes and Public Policies: A Personal Impression." In *Mackenzie King: Widening the Debate*, John English and J. O. Stubbs, eds., Toronto: Macmillan of Canada, pp. 15–29.

Pierson, Paul (2000). "Three Worlds of Welfare State Research." *Comparative Political Studies*, 33, 6/7, pp. 791–821.

Piven, Francis F. and R. A. Cloward (1971). *Regulating the Poor*. New York: Vintage.

——— (1977). *Poor People's Movements: Why They Succeed, How They Fail*. New York: Pantheon.

Poen, Monty M. (1979). *Harry S. Truman versus the Medical Lobby*. Columbia: University of Missouri Press.

Polsby, Nelson W. (1984). *Political Innovation in America: The Politics of Policy Initiation*. New Haven: Yale University Press.

Population Reference Bureau (1995). "1995 World Population Data Sheet." Washington, D.C.

Quadagno, Jill (1987). "Theories of the Welfare State." *Annual Review of Sociology*, 13: 109–28.

——— (1994). *The Color of Welfare: How Racism Undermined the War on Poverty*. New York: Oxford University Press.

Ragin, Charles C. (1987). *The Comparative Method: Moving beyond Qualitative and Quantitative Strategies*. Berkeley: University of California Press.

Ragin, Charles C., Susan E. Mayer, and Kriss A. Drass (1984). "Assessing Discrimination: A Boolean Approach." *American Sociological Review*, 49: 221–34.

Richardson, J. E. (1973). *Patterns of Australian Federalism*. Research Monograph No. 1, Centre for Research on Federal Financial Relations, Canberra: Australian National University Press.

Roe, Jill, ed. (1976). *Social Policy in Australia: Some Perspectives 1901–1975*. Melbourne: Cassell Australia Limited.

Rose, Joseph B. and Gary N. Chaison (1996). "Linking Union Density and Union Effectiveness: The North American Experience." *Industrial Relations*, 35, 1 (January), pp. 78–105.

Ross, Lloyd (1959). "Australian Trade Unionism in the Twentieth Century: A Historical Survey." In *Trade Unions in Australia*, John Wilkes and S. E. Benson, eds., Sydney: Angus & Robertson, pp. 1–46.

Rowan, Richard L. and Herbert R. Northrup (1968). *Readings in Labor Economics and Labor Relations*. Homewood, Ill.: Irwin.

Rubin, Alissa J. (1993). "With Health Overhaul on Stage, PACs Want Front Row Seat." *Congressional Quarterly Weekly Report*, July 31, pp. 2052–54.

Ruggie, Mary (1996). *Realignments in the Welfare State: Health Policy in the United States, Britain, and Canada*. New York: Columbia University Press.

Rush, Benjamin (1787). Quoted in *The Price of Union* by Herbert Agar, Boston: Houghton Mifflin, 1966, pp. 36–37.

Sawer, Geoffrey (1983). "The Constitutional Crisis of Australian Federalism." In *Australian Federalism: Future Tense*, Allan Patience and Jeffrey Scott, eds., Melbourne: Oxford University Press, pp. 94–106.

——— (1988). *The Australian Constitution*. Canberra: Australian Government. Public Service.

Sax, Sidney (1984). *A Strife of Interests: Politics and Policies in Australian Health Services*. Sydney: Allen & Unwin.

——— (1990). *Health Care Choices and the Public Purse*. Sydney: Allen & Unwin.

Schachner, Robert (1990). *The Worker's Paradise? Robert Schachner's Letters from Australia 1906–07*. John Lack, Frederik Ohles, and Jurgen Tampke, eds. Parkville, Victoria: University of Melbourne.

Scotton, R. B. (1980). "Health Insurance: Medibank and After." In *Public Expenditures and Social Policy in Australia, Volume II: The First Fraser Years, 1976–78*, R. B. Scotton and Helen Ferber, eds., Melbourne: Longman Cheshire, pp. 175–219.

Seligman, Adam (1987). "The Failure of Socialism in the United States: A Reconsideration." In *Centre Formation, Protest Movements, and Class Structure in Europe and the United States* by S.N. Eisenstadt, L. Roniger, and A. Seligman, London: Pinter, 1987, pp. 90–117.

Shaw, A. G. L. (1955). *The Story of Australia*. London: Faber & Faber.

Sherman, Mark (2004). "Call for Probe into Medicare Estimate Grows." Associated Press; printed in *The Houston Chronicle*, March 17, 3A.

Shortt, S. E. D. (1983–84). "The Canadian Hospital in the Nineteenth Century: An Historiographic Lament." *Journal of Canadian Studies*, 18, 4, pp. 3–14.

Skidmore, Max J. (1970). *Medicare and the American Rhetoric of Reconciliation*. University: University of Alabama Press.

Skocpol, Theda (1984). "Emerging Agendas and Recurrent Strategies in Historical Sociology." In *Vision and Method in Historical Sociology*, Theda Skocpol, ed., New York: Cambridge University Press, pp. 356–91.

——— (1996). *Boomerang: Clinton's Health Security Effort and the Turn against Government in U.S. Politics*. New York: Norton.

Skocpol, Theda and Edwin Amenta (1986). "States and Social Policies." *Annual Review of Sociology*, 12:131–57.

Smith, Rodney and Michael Wearing (1987). "Do Australians Want the Welfare State?" *Politics*, 22, 2, November, pp. 55–65.

Sorensen, Aage B. (2000). "Toward a Sounder Basis for Class Analysis." *American Journal of Sociology*, 105, 6, pp. 1523–58. (See also following comments by John Goldthorpe and Erik O. Wright, pp. 1559–82.)

Stanfield, J. Ron (1979). "Phenomena and Epiphenomena in Economics." *Journal of Economic Issues*, 13, 4, December, pp. 885–98.

Starr, Paul (1982). *The Social Transformation of American Medicine*. New York: Basic Books.

Starr, Paul and Ellen Immergut (1987). "Health Care and the Boundaries of Politics." In *Changing Boundaries of the Political: Essays on the Evolving Balance between the State and Society, Public and Private in Europe*, Charles S. Maier, ed., 1987, pp. 221–54.

Steinmo, Sven and Jon Watts (1995). "It's the Institutions, Stupid! Why Comprehensive National Health Insurance Always Fails in America." *Journal of Health Politics, Policy and Law*, 20: 329–72.

Stone, Deborah A. (1993). "The Struggle for the Soul of Health Insurance." In *The Politics of Health Care Reform: Lessons from the Past, Prospects for the Future*, James A. Morone and Gary S. Belkin, eds., Durham: Duke University Press, 1994, pp. 26–56.

Sutcliffe, J. T. (1921). *A History of Trade Unionism in Australia*. Workers' Educational Association Series No. 3. Melbourne: MacMillan of Australia.

Sutherland, Tracy (1997). "Rich Can Duck Medicare Rise with $335 in Private Cover." *The Weekend Australian*, June 14–15, p 10.

Taft, Philip (1964). *Organized Labor in American History*. New York: Harper & Row.

Taylor, Malcolm G. (1978). *Health Insurance and Canadian Public Policy: The Seven Decisions That Created the Canadian Health Insurance System*. Montreal: McGill-Queen's University Press.

——— (1990). *Insuring National Health Care: The Canadian Experience*. Chapel Hill: University of North Carolina Press.

Thelen, Kathleen and Sven Steinmo (1992). "Historical Institutionalism in Comparative Politics." In *Structuring Politics: Historical Institutionalism in Comparative Analysis*, Sven Steinmo, Kathleen Thelen, and Frank Longstreth, eds., New York: Cambridge University Press, 1992, pp. 1–32.

Thorburn, Hugh G. (1985). *Interest Groups in the Canadian Federal System*. Toronto: University of Toronto Press.

Tilly, Charles (1984). *Big Structures, Large Processes, and Huge Comparisons*. New York: Sage.

Troy, Leo and Neil Sheflin (1985). *U.S. Union Sourcebook*. Industrial Relations Date and Information Services. West Orange, N.J.: Donnelley & Sons.

U.S. Bureau of the Census (1988). *Statistical Abstract of the United States: 1988* (110th edition). Washington, D.C.: U.S. Government Printing Office.

Van Loon, Richard J. and Michael S. Whittington (1976). *The Canadian Political System: Environment, Structure and Process*. Toronto: McGraw-Hill Ryerson.

Vayda, Eugene and Raisa B. Deber (1992). "The Canadian Health-Care System: A Developmental Overview." In *Canadian Health Care and the State: A Century of Evolution*, C. David Naylor, ed., Montreal: McGill-Queen's University Press, pp. 125–40.

Walker, Harold Lloyd (1978). "The A.M.A. and Compulsory N.H.I.: The Molding of Public Opinion, 1920–1965." Ph.D. thesis. University of Texas at Austin.

Weinberg, Adam S. and Kenneth A. Gould (1993). "Public Participation in Environmental Regulatory Conflicts: Treading through the Possibilities and Pitfalls." *Law and Policy*, 15, 2 (April), 139–67.

Weir, Margaret and Theda Skocpol (1983). "State Structures and Social Keynesianism: Responses to the Great Depression in Sweden and the United States." *International Journal of Comparative Sociology*, 24, 1–2, 4–27.

——— (1986). "State Structures and the Possibilities for 'Keynesian' Responses to the Great Depression in Sweden, Britain, and the United States." In *Bringing the State Back In*, Peter B. Evans, Dietrich Rueschemeye, and Theda Skocpol, eds., Cambridge: Cambridge University Press, pp. 107–63.

Weisman, Jonathan (2004). "Deficit Hurtling to Record High; Shortfall May Be $477 Billion." *The Washington Post*; reprinted in *The Houston Chronicle*, January 27, 1A.

White, Joseph (1995). "The Horses and the Jumps: Comments on the Health Care Reform Steeplechase." *Journal of Health Politics, Policy and Law*, 20:373–83.

Wilensky, H. (1975). *The Welfare State and Equality: Structural and Ideological Roots of Public Expenditures*. Berkeley: University of California Press.

Wilensky, H., Gregory Luebbert, Susan Reed Hahn, and Adrienne Jamieson (1987). "Comparative Social Policy: Theories, Methods, Findings." In *Comparative Policy Research: Learning from Experience*, Meinolf Dierkes, Hans Weiler, and Ariane Berthoin Antal, eds., New York: St. Martin's, pp. 381–457.

Young, Judith (1992). "'A Necessary Nuisance': Social Class and Parental Visiting Rights at Toronto's Hospital for Sick Children 1930–1970." In *Canadian Health Care and the State: A Century of Evolution*, C. David Naylor, ed., Montreal: McGill-Queen's University Press, pp. 85–103.

Zieger, Robert H. (1986). *American Workers, American Unions, 1920–1985*. Baltimore: Johns Hopkins University Press.

Index

access, xxii, 91–93, 98, 126–27,
131–32, 146
Australian, 39, 42, 46, 56
Canadian, 9, 16, 21, 30, 111
United States, 1, 59, 83, 85, 113,
115
Adjustment Commission, 67
Alberta, 10, 12, 16–17, 20, 22, 26–28,
32
Alford, Robert R., xxvii
Amenta, Edwin, xii, xxv, 99
American Association for Labor Legis-
lation (AALL), 65–66
American Federation of Labor, (AFL),
13–14, 64, 67–69
American Federation of Labor and
Congress of Industrial Organiza-
tions, (AFL-CIO), 14, 80
American Hospital Association, 71
American labor tactics, 14
American Medical Association, (AMA),
23, 66, 68, 72–76, 81, 113–15. *See
also* organized medicine
American Public Health Association,
77
Anderson, Odin W., 66, 71–72, 74–76
arbitration, 47, 53, 56, 68
Arcadia, 5–6
Articles of Confederation, 61–62
assisted immigration, 36
Australian Labor Party, 33, 39, 42–58,
70, 112–13, 128–29

Australian Medical Association,
(AMA), 33, 38–47, 51, 146. *See
also* organized medicine
Austria, xxviii, 95

bank panic, 64
Banting, Keith, x, xii–xiii, xxiv, 29–30
Battle of the Clubs, 37
benevolent societies, 34–35
Blendon, Robert J., xi
block grants, 80
blockage, 55, 59, 86–87, 89, 117
Blue Cross, 20, 69, 71–72
Blue Shield, 69, 72
boolean algebra, xxii, 100, 138
Britain, xxvi–xxvii, 40–41
and Canada, 9–10, 13, 22, 30
and Australia, 34, 37, 61
and the United States, 86
See also England
British Columbia, 10, 12, 15–16, 20,
22, 26–27, 32
British House of Commons, 60
British North America Act, 9, 11
bulk billing, 47
Bush, George, 81–82
Business Week, 77

California, 69, 73
Canada Health Act, 29
Canadian Congress of Labor, (CCL),
14–15

Canadian constitution, 11
Canadian Labor Congress (CLC), 14
Canadian Medical Association, (CMA), 23–24, 26. *See also* organized medicine
capitation, 9
Carter, Jimmy, 80–82
Catholic Church, 6, 95
central state structures, xii
centralization, xvii, 62
Chamber of Commerce, 23
charity, 8–9, 34–35
Charity Aid Act, 8
chemists, 36
Chifley, Ben, 42–44
choice of nations, x, xviii, xxiii–xxix, 2
Christian democratic parties, xxv, xxvi
civil conscription, 25, 43
class power, xviii–xix, 92–94, 107–9, 115–17, 146
Clinton, Bill, 82
Clinton, Hillary, 83
Cloward, R.A., xiv
Cold War, 74
College of Physicians and Surgeons, 22, 25. *See also* organized medicine
commercial insurance, xxix, 66
Committee for National Health Insurance, 77
Committee on Economic Security (CES), 68
Common Form of Agreement, 38
Commonwealth Constitution Act, 37
community-based rates, 83
comparative studies, xi, xvii, 120–21
comparative historical methods, ix, xix–xxiii, 2, 97, 111, 120–21
compromise
  Australian, 52, 113, 131
  Canadian, 109
  United States, 59, 76, 78, 80, 83, 114, 130
compulsory insurance, 66
confederation, 8–11, 14, 61–62, 86

Confederation of National Trade Unions (CNTU), 14
configurations, xvi, 101–5, 132–33, 138–40, 146–47
Congress (U.S.), xii, 117, 123–25
  and health care policy, 67–68, 72–75, 78–83, 85–87, 89
Congress of Industrial Organizations (CIO), 13, 14, 68, 69, 80
Congress of the Confederation, 62
Congressional Budget and Anti-Impoundment Act, 79
Congressional Budget Office, 79
congressional committees, 84
conjunctural causation, xxi–xxiv, xxix, 97, 107–8, 119
Conservative Party, 11–12. *See also* Progressive Conservative Party
conservative welfare states, xxviii
conservatives, xiii, 12, 44, 62, 74, 83–84
constitutional amendment, 18, 33, 43
constitutional authority, 42, 137
Constitutional Convention, 63
Consumer Price Index, 83
contracts, 35, 37–38, 51, 60, 67–68, 71
convergence theory, x
Cooperative Commonwealth Federation (CCF), 12, 15–26, 30, 32, 70, 86–87, 111–12. *See also* New Democratic Party
cooperatives, 64, 71
corporate structures, 54
costs, xxii, 1, 4, 92, 95, 126
  Australian, 41–42, 44–47, 49–50, 56
  Canadian, 18–20, 25, 29–30, 112
  United States, xvi, 66, 70–71, 76–83, 85, 114
  See also medical inflation
cost-sharing, 22, 48
Cottage Hospital and Medical Care plan, 17
court arbitration, 47
Coxie's army, 64
craft unions, 12, 64

cultural theory, x, xi, xviii
currency, 62

Dahl, Robert A., xi, xiii
Declaration of Independence, 61
decommodification, xvii, xxvii–xxviii,
    78, 92–93, 127, 145–46
decommodifying programs, 50–52, 96,
    104, 136–37, 143, 147
  criteria, 100, 126–32
  nondecommodifying programs, xvi,
    83, 102–3, 110
democracy, 25, 62, 65, 87, 92–93, 119
democratic class struggle, xiv, xvi, 53,
    91, 96
Democratic Party, xiii, 30, 88
  and health policy, xv, 72–73, 75–76,
    80, 82, 94, 115
  and labor, 64–65, 67, 70, 87
democratic state, xiv, xxviii, 92
Democrats. *See* Democratic Party
Denmark, xxviii, 95
Depression, xv, 16–18, 37, 39, 61–62,
    67–70, 87
diagnosis-related groups (DRG), 81
direct service insurance, 70–71
division of political power, 55, 63
Domhoff, G. William, 96, 146
dominion-provincial conferences, 19
dualism, xxvii, xxviii, 100, 109, 130–32

efficiency, 63, 87–88, 119
Eisenhower, Dwight D., 75
elderly, 59, 74–76, 95, 114, 128. *See
    also* pensioners
electoral processes, xiii
emergent factors, 134, 136–37, 141
employers, 96
  Australian, 39
  Canadian, 9, 12–13
  United States, 63, 66–68, 70–72, 77,
    79, 82–84
England, 6, 35, 60, 62. *See also* Britain
Employment Retirement Income
    Security Act (ERISA), 79

Esping-Andersen, Gosta, xiv–xv, xxv,
    xxviii, 91–92, 145
European Enlightenment, 61
Evans, Robert, 30
exceptionalism, xvii, xix
  United States, xii, xiv–xv, xxiii, 3, 98,
    115, 117
expression, 100–2, 138–40, 146
extra-billing, xxx, 29

failure of socialism, (U.S.), xiv
farmers' revolts, 62
federal financial leverage, 31, 43, 102,
    104, 108, 115–16, 137
federal power in health field, 101–2,
    105–7, 135–37, 141–43
federalism, xxvii, xxix
federation, xii, 3, 9, 36, 37
Federation des Medecins Specialistes
    du Quebec (FMSQ), 28
fee schedules, 29, 56
fee-for-service, 9, 20, 29, 38, 41–43,
    48–49, 78
Fein, Rashi, x, xxv, 70–72, 75–78, 80,
    124
First Continental Congress, 61
five federal conditions, 30
Florida, 64
Forand, Aime J., 76
Ford, Gerald, 80–81
Fortune, 77
Founding Fathers, 62
France, xxviii, 5–7, 10, 60, 95
Fraser, Malcolm, 49–51
fraternal benefit associations, 64
free hospital experiment, 42, 44, 56,
    130
free hospitalization, 38, 47, 49–50,
    112–13
French Canada, 5–8, 10, 14, 61
friendly societies, 34–38, 40–41, 45
Front de Liberation du Quebec
    (FLQ), 28
Frost, Leslie, 21
Fuchs, Victor, x, xxv

gaps, xvi, 46–47, 59, 81, 85
general practitioners, 41
Germany, xxviii, 95
Ginzberg, Eli, x, xxv
Gompers, Samuel, 66
Gordon, Walter, 28
Gottschalk, Marie, xiv, 70, 73, 78–79, 83–84, 96
Gray, Gwendolyn, xii, xxix, 9, 16–30, 33, 42–51
Green Book Proposals, 18–19
Griffiths, Martha, 77

Hamilton, 12
Hawke, Bob, 50
health financing, 85, 93
health maintenance organization (HMO), 78
health policy legacies, 92–93, 100, 109, 115, 131–32
    Australian health policy, 33–34, 53, 56, 113
    Canadian health policy, 19, 104
    United States health policy, xiv, 74, 76
Health Security Act, 83–84
hearings, 18, 26, 73, 75
herbalists, 36
Hicks, Alexander, xxii, xxv, 133
Hirshfield, Daniel S., xi, 65–66, 69
Hollingsworth, J. Rogers, xiii, 83–84, 124
honorary physicians, 40
Hospital Benefits Act, 44–45
Hospital Insurance and Diagnostic Services Act, 22
hospitalization insurance
    Australian, 49
    Canadian, 20, 30, 111
    United States, 69, 71–72, 74–76, 114
    See also free hospitalization and free hospital experiment
House
    of Commons (Canadian), 17, 28

    of Representatives (Australian), 47–48
    of Representatives (U.S.), 3, 54, 76, 79, 87, 124
    Ways and Means Committee, 75, 95
Howard, John, 52
Huber, Evelyne, xii, xxv, 145

Immergut, Ellen, xii–xiii, 94, 96
indemnity insurance, 70–71
indenture, 60
indirect method of difference, xx–xxi, xxiv, 108
industrial unions, 13, 67
Industrial Workers of the World (IWW), 64
industrialization, x, xxv, 65, 67
Insurance Economic Society, 66
interest groups, xi, 2, 91, 94, 96, 115
    Australian, 54, 58
    Canadian, 18
    United States, 3, 54, 70, 84, 87–89
Italy, xxviii, 95

Johnson, Lyndon, 75, 114
joint sitting, 48

Kaiser, 78
Keep Our Doctors committees, 23
Kennedy, Edward, 77, 88
Kennedy, John F., 75–78, 80, 88, 94, 114
Kerr-Mills, 75–76, 114, 128
Knights of Labor, 13, 64
Korpi, Walter, xiv–xv, 91, 145

labor, 91–92
labor market, xiii, xxviii, 92, 126–27
labor movement, xiv, 96
    Canadian, 12–16, 18, 26, 28
    Australian, 36–37, 112
    United States, xiii–xv, xviii, xxiii, 63–70, 72, 75, 78, 80, 83–89, 98, 118

labor parties, xxx, 95
  Australian, xxvii–xxviii, 37
  Canadian, xxviii, 15
  United States, xv, xxviii, 86, 115, 145
labor party power, 101–2, 104–7, 109,
  116, 135–37, 141–43
Labour-Progressive Party (LPP), 15
Laham, Nicholas, xiii, 77–78, 80–84
legacies, xxvi, 18, 60, 70
  cultural, 5–6
  legislative, 101–2, 104, 116, 135–36,
    141–43
  policy (non-health), xii, xix, xxv,
    xxviii, xxx
  political, xiii, 15, 32, 54, 58, 95–97,
    106–8
  state/provincial, 16, 104, 112
  legitimation, 24, 63, 92–93, 95–96,
    103
  See also health policy legacies
leverage, xii. *See also* federal financial
  leverage
Lewis, John, 68
liberal nations, 94
Liberal Party, 11, 15, 17, 23, 26, 30
liberal welfare states, xxviii, 109
Lipset, Seymour Martin, x, xiii, xxiii,
  xxv, 16, 98
Lower Canada, 7–9

Maioni, Antonia, xiii, xxiv, 17–21,
  26–28, 69–75, 117
majority rule, 58, 92, 96
Manitoba, 10, 12, 16–17, 22
market, xvii
  health care, 42, 51, 91–93
  labor, xxviii, xxx, 13, 67, 83, 91–92
  worker dependence on, xv–xvi,
    xxvii
market-oriented policy, 93, 100
  Australian, 45, 55
  criteria, xv, 100, 126–28, 130–31, 147
  legacies, xxviii, xxx, 131
  legacy (U.S.), xiii, xv, xxvi, 59, 85
Marmor, Theodore R., xi

Marshall, T.H., 92
Marx, Karl, 15, 91
Massachusetts, 61, 63, 69
maternity grant, 37
McConnell, Grant, xi
means test, xxii, 26, 45, 80, 98
means-tested programs, xv, 27, 85
mediating system, 94
Medibank, 46–51, 54, 56, 113, 147
Medicaid, 59, 76, 80–85, 114, 128
medical inflation, 25, 77, 81. *See also*
  costs
medical service, 19, 33–34, 39–40, 42,
  45–46, 71
Medicare
  Australian, 50–53, 56, 113, 128–29,
    147
  Canadian, 5, 24, 28–30, 128–29
  United States, xv–xvi, 74–78, 80–82,
    85, 94–95, 114, 123, 127–30
Medicare Prescription Drug Act, 85,
  114
Menzies, Robert, 45, 47
method of agreement, xx–xxi,
  xxiii–xxiv, 108
Michigan, 69
midwives, 7–8, 36
Mills, John Stuart, xx–xxi, 95, 114,
  123, 128
Mills, Wilbur, 75–76, 78
Misra, Joya, xxv
momentum, 16, 59, 70, 84
Montreal, 5, 7, 12
Morone, James A., xiii
multiparty system, 101–2, 104–8, 118,
  136–37, 141–43
multiparty systems, xii, 94, 116
multiple conjunctural causation,
  107–8, 119
multiple independent causation,
  xx–xxi, xxix, 97, 107–8

National Association of Manufacturers
  (NAM), 66
National Governors' Conference, 77

National Health and Pensions Insurance Bill, 39
national health insurance (NHI), xxii, 91–118, 132–35, 141–42, 145
  Australian, 33, 52–58
  Canadian, 5, 12, 18–19, 25–32
  comparative, xix, xxviii–xxix
  typology, 126–32
  United States, ix, xiii, xvi, xxiii, 59, 70–88
  See also public health insurance
National Health Service, 22
National Health Service Act, 44
National Insurance Bill, 39
National War Labor Board, 68
National Welfare Fund, 43
Native Americans, 6
natural rights of man, 61
Navarro, Vicente, ix–xi, xiv, xv, xxiii, xxvi, 98
negative cases, xxi–xxiv, 98–99, 105, 108, 132
New Brunswick, 9, 10, 22
New Democratic Party (NDP), xxvii, 15–16, 24, 26–32, 86–87, 112
New France, 5–7
New Protection, 37
New South Wales, 33–38, 48, 51, 112
New York, 6, 63–64, 69, 75–76
New Zealand, xxvi–xxvii
Newfoundland, 10, 17, 20
Nixon, Richard, 76, 78–79, 114
noncooperation, 39, 113
non-Labor, 33, 37–40, 43–58, 127, 128
Northwest Territories, 10
Norway, xxviii, 95
Nova Scotia, 5–6, 8–10, 22

official formulary, 43
Olsen, Gregg M., x–xiv, 12, 29–30, 145
Ontario, 8–10, 12–15, 17, 19–22, 26–28
optimal care, 93
organized medicine, 87, 137
  Canadian, 17, 20, 22–29

See also the American, Australian and Canadian Medical Associations
Orloff, Ann Shola, xix, xxiii–xxiv, 98–99
outpatient treatment, 34
O'Connor, Julia S., xxiv, 145, 146

Pampel, Fred C., xi, xxv, 145
Parliament
  Australian, 47, 54
  British, 9, 37, 61–62
  Canadian, 13, 15, 22, 27, 31, 112
  Swedish, 94
parliamentary system, xxvi, 12, 14, 32–33, 58–59, 62, 123
Parti Quebecois, 12
patterns
  causal, xvi, xxi, 97, 99, 103, 107–8, 138, 140, 147. *See also* configurations
  policy, xxvii
  and variable choices, 120, 133–34
pensioners, 45, 49, 52, 113. *See also* elderly
Pharmaceutical Benefits Act, 43
Philadelphia, 63–64
Piven, Francis F., xiv
pluralist political dynamics, xi
pluralist theory, xi, 96
polarization, 33, 53–54, 59
policy types, 128, 130
political action committees, 69
political costs, xix, 145
political institutional factors, xxx, 96, 108, 115–17, 137
political institutional theories, xii
political institutions, xvi, xviii, 91, 93–95, 116
  Canadian, 10, 31
  Australian, 53–54
  United States, 62, 87, 117, 119, 123
Political Labor League, 38
Polsby, Nelson W., xi
Populist movement, 71
Portugal, 60

positive cases, xx–xxi, xxiii, 98, 108
possible causal factors, xxiii–xxv, xxviii,
    97–98
power, x–xii, 2–3, 115, 146
    Australian, 33, 37, 39, 43, 46, 55–57,
        104–5
    Canadian, 11–12, 15, 22–23, 27, 30,
        104, 111
    resources factors, xviii, xxx, 91,
        107–9, 115–17, 120
    resources theory, xiv–xvi, 53, 96, 145
    United States, 3, 62–63, 79, 87–88,
        105–6, 116–19, 121
    See also class power, federal power,
        and labor party power
prepayment plans, 70–72
president, xii, 54–55, 63, 78–79, 85–86,
    123–25
President's Commission on the Health
    Needs of the Nation, 74
Prince Edward Island, 9, 22
private administration of public pro-
    grams, 22, 24
private care, 17, 34–35, 41–42, 46, 50
private doctors, 7, 37
private fees, 38
private health care industry, 74, 80, 88,
    127
private hospitals, 40–41, 45, 48, 57
private insurance, 23–4, 41–42, 51,
    69–72, 80
    companies, xxx, 48, 50, 83, 126
    components of Australian public
        programs, 46–47, 50, 113
    components of public programs, 93,
        100, 126–31
    components of U.S. public pro-
        grams, xv, 75, 85, 114
    coverage, 21, 75, 135, 137
private patients, 9, 41, 47
private practice, 29, 35, 37, 40–42
private sector interests, xiii, 16, 49,
    56–57, 67, 92
private welfare state, 96, 146
Progressive Party, 11, 15

propertyless, 63
proportional representation, xxx, 94,
    105, 135, 137
public benefits, 50, 92, 130
public clinics, 37, 43
public control of costs, 29, 79, 83, 92
public funding of elections, 58
public health, 10, 37–38, 65, 69, 77
    insurance advocates, 69, 75
    policy, 57, 74–75, 124–32, 136, 143
    services, 9, 38, 46
public health insurance, 93, 100
    Australian, 46, 49, 51–52, 113
    Canadian, 21, 23–24, 26, 32, 111–12
    United States, 3, 59, 76, 80, 85, 118
    See also national health insurance
public hospitals, 7, 33–35, 38, 40–42,
    44, 48
public policy, xv–xvi, 121
public-private mix, xxvii–xxix, 93,
    125–26, 137, 146
public relations campaigns, 73, 84,
    88–89
public support, x–xi
    Australian, 53, 58
    Canadian, 5, 17, 21–22, 30
    United States, 75, 82–84, 94, 114
public wards, 44, 45

Quadagno, Jill, x–xiii, xxv
qualitative, ix, xvii–xix, xxvii
qualitative comparative analysis
    (QCA), xxii, xxx–xxxi, 97–101,
    115–16, 132–43
Quebec, 5–7, 9, 12–14, 19–22, 27–28,
    32
Queensland, 36, 42

radicalism, 14, 67
Ragin, Charles C., xix–xxv, 100, 107,
    133, 139
Ralliement des Creditistes, 12
Reagan, Ronald, 81, 83
Red River colony, 10
redistribution, xv–xviii, xxvi, 50, 83

referendums, 37, 54
reform movement, 65
Republicans. *See* Republican Party
Republican Party, 67, 73, 75, 77–79,
    81, 84–86, 88
residual programs, 100, 131
responsibility, xxx, 92
    Australian, 38, 58
    Canadian, 8, 19, 25, 29
    United States, 55, 68, 81, 84
responsible party government, xiii,
    xxviii–xxx, 11, 62, 86–87, 94
Reuther, Walter, 70, 77
Revolutionary War, 61
right to organize, 63, 65
Roosevelt, Franklin D., 67, 69, 94, 114
Rowell-Sirois Royal Commission on
    Dominion-Provincial Relations,
    18
royal commissions, 18, 26, 39, 112
Royal Commission on Health Services,
    26
rural cooperative movement, 16

salaries, 7–8, 47, 51
Saskatchewan, 10, 12, 15–16, 19–27,
    32, 111
Saskatchewan Association of Rural
    Municipalities, 20
Saskatchewan Citizens for Medicare,
    24
Saskatchewan Hospitals Service Plan,
    20
school health services, 37
Second Continental Congress, 61
Senate
    Australian, 47–50, 54, 105, 113
    Canadian, 28
    United States, xiii, 3, 54–55, 63, 73,
        78–79, 87, 124
sessional payments, 48, 51
single theory approaches, xvi
Skocpol, Theda, xii–xiii, xx, xxiii, xxv,
    83–84, 98
social class, xv, xvii–xviii, 35
Social Credit Party, 12, 32

social democratic, xi, 3, 26, 55, 95, 120
    Australian factors, 109
    dynamics, xviii, 91
    Canadian factors, 26, 104, 116
    parties, xxv, 12, 24, 94, 116
    regimes, xxviii
    theory, xiv, 145. *See* power resources
        theory
    U.S. factors, 117–18
social right, 92
Social Security, xv–xvi, 68, 74–76, 114
Socialist Labor Party, 65
Sorensen, Aage, 91
South Australia, 36, 48
Spain, 60
specialists, xvii, 25, 28, 41, 48, 51
St. Laurent, Louis, 21
Starr, Paul, ix, xi, xiii, 69–80
State Children's Health Insurance Pro-
    gram (SCHIP), 84–85, 114
state constitutions, 61–62
state medical societies, 66, 72
Steinmo, Sven, ix, xii–xiii, xxiii, 94, 98
Stephens, John D.
Stone, Deborah A., xiii, xxvi
stratification, xvii, xxvii, 146
subsidies, 100, 131
    Australian, 34–35, 44, 50, 52, 70,
        113, 118
    Canadian, 8, 22, 70, 111, 118
    United States, 74, 85
suffrage, xiii, 63
Supreme Court (U.S.), 69, 89
Sweden, xxviii, 94–95
Sydney, 34–36, 41

Taft-Hartley Act, 79
Tasmania, 36, 40, 42, 48
taxes, 6, 19–20, 38, 49, 61, 81–83
Taylor, Malcolm, 8–9, 17–28
territories, 10, 62
theoretical approaches, x, xii, xvi
theoretical premises, xviii
third parties, xiii, 11–12, 31, 69
Three Worlds of Welfare Capitalism,
    xxvii

Tilly, Charles, xx
Toronto, 12, 13
trade practices legislation, 47
Trades and Labor Congress of Canada
    (TLCC), 14–15
transported convicts, 33
Truman, Harry, 72–74, 82, 94, 114
truth tables, 103, 138, 140
two-party systems, 116
two-tier systems, 93
typology, 126, 128, 130, 132

unemployed, 61, 64, 67, 72, 93
uninsured, 21, 45, 78, 82–84, 92, 126
Union Hospital Districts, 16
Union Nationale, 12
United Kingdom. *See* Britain
United Mine Workers, 68
universality, xxii, 29, 98
Upper Canada, 8

Vancouver Island, 10
veterans, 52, 66
veto points, 101–2, 107, 115–16, 121,
    134–37, 141–43
    Australian, 54, 105, 109, 113
    Canadian, 31–32, 104, 109, 112, 116
    United States, 84, 86, 88, 105–6,
        109, 115–18, 121

Victoria, 36, 38
Virginia, 60
voluntary insurance, 23–28, 41, 128

Wagner Health Bill, 68
Watts, Jon, ix, xii–xiii, xxiii, 94, 98
Weir, Margaret, xiii
welfare state, xxv, 91, 95–96, 118,
    120–21, 146
    Australian, 38–39, 56, 58, 102–3
    Canadian, 28–29, 102–3
    theories, ix–xviii, 3, 145–46
    types, xxvii–xxviii
    United States, 76, 96, 102–3
Western Australia, 36
White, Joseph, xiii–xiv, xxvi
Whitlam, Gough, 46–47
window of opportunity, 106
Wisconsin, 69
working class, xiv–xv, xviii–xix, xxv,
    xxvii, 2, 91–96, 145–46
    Australian, 35, 53, 58, 87, 116
    Canadian, 16, 87
    United States, xi, xvi, xviii, 3, 70,
        87–89, 145
Working Men's parties, 64
working-class agitation, xiv
World War I, 38, 65–67, 113
World War II, 16, 42, 68–69, 112